facts

The pill

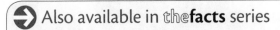

Also available in the**facts** series

thefacts

The pill

SEVENTH EDITION

JOHN GUILLEBAUD
ANNE MACGREGOR

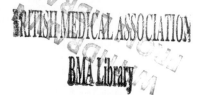

OXFORD
UNIVERSITY PRESS

OXFORD

UNIVERSITY PRESS

Great Clarendon Street, Oxford OX2 6DP

Oxford University Press is a department of the University of Oxford.
It furthers the University's objective of excellence in research, scholarship,
and education by publishing worldwide in

Oxford New York

Auckland Cape Town Dar es Salaam Hong Kong Karachi
Kuala Lumpur Madrid Melbourne Mexico City Nairobi
New Delhi Shanghai Taipei Toronto

With offices in

Argentina Austria Brazil Chile Czech Republic France Greece
Guatemala Hungary Italy Japan Poland Portugal Singapore
South Korea Switzerland Thailand Turkey Ukraine Vietnam

Oxford is a registered trade mark of Oxford University Press
in the UK and in certain other countries

Published in the United States
by Oxford University Press Inc., New York

British Library Cataloguing in Publication Data

Data available

Typeset in Plantin
by Cepha Imaging Pvt. Ltd., Bangalore, India
Printed in Great Britain by Ashford Colour Press, Gosport, Hampshire

ISBN 978-0-19-956576-4

10 9 8 7 6 5 4 3 2 1

John Guillebaud MA, FRCSEd, FRCOG, Hon FFSRH, Hon FCOG(SA) Professor Emeritus of Family Planning and Reproductive Health, University College, London, was raised in East Africa, his parents living in what was then called Ruanda-Urundi. He is now Emeritus Professor of Family Planning and Reproductive Health, University College London. He was the world's first gynaecologist and vasectomy surgeon to be given a personal chair in that specialty. He worked for 25 years as a consultant at the Hospital for Women Soho which merged to become the United Elizabeth Garrett Anderson Hospital and was also the Medical Director of the Margaret Pyke Family Planning Centre. He continues in clinical work at the Churchill Hospital's Elliot-Smith Vasectomy Clinic in Oxford. He acts periodically as a consultant to the World Health Organization (WHO) and other national and international bodies in the reproductive health field. He originated the Environment Time Capsule Project at www.ecotimecapsule.com, is Trustee of TASKwh (Towards African Solutions through Knowledge for Women's Health), Co-Chair of www.populationands ustainability.org, and Chair of Planet 21 (www.peopleandplanet.net).

Anne MacGregor MD, MFSRH, MICR, DIPM Honorary Senior Clinical Lecturer, Research Centre for Neuroscience within the Institute of Cell and Molecular Science, Barts and the London School of Medicine and Dentistry. Anne works in sexual and reproductive healthcare at St Bartholomew's Hospital and is an Instructing Doctor and CRQ Convener for the Faculty of Sexual and Reproductive Healthcare of the Royal College of Obstetricians and Gynaecologists. She is also Clinical Research Director at the City of London Migraine Clinic, an independent medical charity, and Honorary Senior Clinical Lecturer at the Research Centre for Neuroscience within the Institute of Cell and Molecular Science, Barts and the London School of Medicine and Dentistry, London.

Foreword to the seventh edition

For this latest fully updated edition, the publisher and I, John Guillebaud (JG), warmly welcome Dr Anne MacGregor (AM) as second author. She provides a fresh perspective as a woman and as a doctor with a special interest and experience in neurology, sex hormones and all aspects of reproductive healthcare.

To explain the book's origins before its first edition in 1980 (with JG then as sole author), I need to go back further, to 1959. I was then a teenage second-year medical student and attended an informal lecture of the St John's Cambridge Medical Society. The biologist Dr Colin Bertram, way ahead of his time, discussed the daunting problems that were bound to be posed by ever-increasing human numbers in the meeting of human needs, along with the needs of the many other species whose habitats humans inevitably alter or destroy. There were no visual aids, the audience was small, but the lecture changed the course of my adult life.

I decided back then that voluntary, available and accessible contraception for all couples on earth, is crucial: not just for them but for the larger world. First, it helps (along with other measures) to prevent efforts to relieve future poverty and suffering being overwhelmed by new arrivals: by ensuring that women are able to fulfil their reproductive right to plan their families. Think of just one example, India, where despite apparent increasing wealth much poverty persists. Although average family size has reduced considerably in that great country compared with 50 years ago, there are every three weeks over a million extra mostly poor people to be housed, fed and educated. Secondly, it is necessary for environmental sustainability, though again not sufficient on its own (see the Figure below, it is like two sides of a coin)[1].

---

[1] *'The very greenest energy is the energy you don't use'* The greatest energy use is by the rich (or minority) world. And it is absolutely crucial that all over-consumers reduce their consumption. But of course as global population increases and as poverty is reduced (as it should be) through development, world energy consumption and therefore CO_2 emissions must increase. As Professor Chris Rapley, (Director, Science Museum London) said *'An absent human has a zero [carbon] footprint'* [Image courtesy of www.PopulationandSustainability.org]

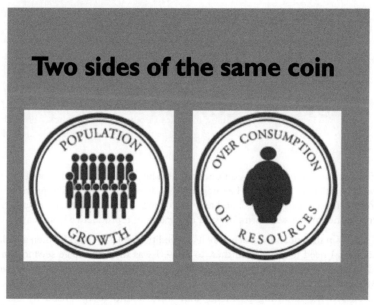

Environmental sustainability means attending to both issues, they are two sides of the same coin.

I therefore came to think, back then and now, that the pill and injection and IUD are at least as important for achieving long-term sustainability on a finite planet as is, say, riding bicycles or properly insulating our homes and workplaces.... Indeed later, in 1994, I ensured that contraceptives were placed in the Kew environment time capsule www.ecotimecapsule.com, alongside the more obvious items like one of my cycle pumps and an ozone-friendly aerosol can.

Dr Bertram highlighted a special responsibility of the medical profession, since it was we who, through amazing medical advances starting around 150 years ago, unintentionally created a problem through the new imbalance between world death-rates and birth-rates. For thousands of years with almost no effective contraception, a couple's normal sex life led, as it always can, to large families of 7-8 or more. Yet, since prior to the mid-1800s most of what doctors did was at best placebos and at worst damaging (eg blood-letting), only a fraction over two children in each average family would survive to be parents for the next generation. So the world population grew slowly. Then came public health measures and later antibiotics with the result that we had hugely improved "death control"; and hence survival of far more children to parenthood, and lower death rates for the adult population too. Since those days we have had an unprecedented almost sevenfold rise in the human population to very nearly 7,000 million, and this increases by about 78 million per year.

Therefore each week now world population goes up by what amounts to a huge city, appearing somewhere, for 1.5 million people – using land and obviously creating more greenhouse gases. Meanwhile of course the planet itself has grown no larger, and three-quarters of it continues to be salt water, with half of the rest being desert, ice, mountain – or rainforest, though sadly too much of that is going or gone.

Feeling responsible after Dr Bertram's talk for my profession's collective failure to make available the balancing measure of contraception quickly enough, I therefore took all the necessary career steps to make reproductive health my own medical specialty.

In this century, impeccable science is telling us that humankind's collective emissions of greenhouse gases are now threatening irreversible climate change. Furthermore the Living Planet Report (www.panda.org/news_facts/publications/living_planet_report/index.cfm) shows that humans are already over-shooting the planet's total bio-capacity (meaning over-use beyond possible supply of fresh water, croplands, fisheries, and forests) and that "by midcentury humanity's demand on nature will be twice the biosphere's productive capacity". According to their data this means that by 2050, the projected population of 9400 million will be trying to use two planets' worth of bio-capacity. With no second planet available, sustainability may be forced on us. Humankind faces the real possibility of a massive cull by Nature in the second half of this century through violence (often fighting over the last few gallons of oil and fresh water), starvation and disease – all worsened by climate change disasters such as hurricanes, floods, droughts, and rising sea levels. As well as moving to low carbon economies as a matter of urgency it must help if reproductive health services, and in particular, the means for voluntary family planning, are made universally accessible.

Making these two essential actions a priority is the ultimate human challenge. Neither is easy, since we in the minority world must admit we have become 'addicted' to our profligate use of energy, and the way of life it has made possible. And the second action has been seriously hindered by the legacy of coercive programmes in some developing countries, notably India in the 1970s and more recently China. Yet coercion is as unnecessary as it is wrong. Allowing for known factors like high child mortality and the need to have children to look after them in old age, my own discussions with women in my birth-continent of Africa, backed by major demographic survey work, show that very many women really want to have smaller families than their normal sex-lives, in the absence of family planning, force them to have – unplanned. Moreover about a third of the nearly 600,000 who die in the world through pregnancy and childbirth, tragically (it's as though a jumbo jet of pregnant women crashes every 6 hours!) and what is worse avoidably, are being killed by a pregnancy they did not wish to conceive. So it is vital, for many reasons way beyond conserving the environment, to address the many barriers to contraception for millions and meet the unmet need for that rights-based choice. Important barriers are lack of information through better education and the media (see www. populationmedia.com), misinformation, simple unavailability of the methods and men preventing access. There are more.

If the world were run by biologists, like Dr Bertram, rather than economists … would we have realised sooner that, for humans like any species in a finite habitat, population matters? Like most people, I love children, indeed people tell me I am besotted by our two grandchildren Isabella (2) and Jamie (6 months). But should we not all from now on, anywhere in the world, consider the future when we decide our family size?

"We have not inherited the earth from our grandparents, we have borrowed it from our grandchildren" (a quote from Kashmir)

[If you are interested to learn more on these issues, please visit all the websites given here also www.populationeducation.org to obtain the amazing DVD "Population dots"]

From that long preamble you now know why, when OUP asked me in 1978 to write a book about the Pill for a general readership, I accepted with alacrity. An equally important reason for the book was to counter a common accusation against doctors: that we knew a lot of worrying facts about the pill, but were not prepared to share them in case the knowledge interfered with women docilely taking their tablets! I decided to attempt to convey virtually everything I knew about the method, bad news and good, and then let people make up their own minds: 'here are the facts, now you decide.'

In this seventh edition, which has been helpfully abridged (mainly by AM) and fully revised, Anne and I believe that we have once again produced the most comprehensive up-to-date handbook on the Pill for non-specialists, in context with other methods of contraception. With each new edition, two principles have been consistently applied: accuracy about what is known, and honesty about what is still unknown—despite much more money being spent researching the safety of the pill than was ever spent on its development.

Any fair-minded reader of this book will find that the facts still support the view that the pill *is* a reasonable option for fully informed women—but certainly not for all. It is important to insist on sufficient information to weigh up and choose between all your options.

As Gwyneth Guillebaud wrote in the foreword to an earlier edition *"Knowledge gives you power"*—empowerment to exercise your own judgement and your human rights about any means that you choose, allowing you to have control over your own fertility. You are the boss!

John Guillebaud & Anne MacGregor

May 2009

Contents

Part 3
Taking the pill

Abbreviations

(See also Glossary)

AIDS	acquired immune deficiency syndrome
BBD	benign breast disease
BMI	body mass index—see Glossary
BTB	breakthrough bleeding
CIN	cervical intraepithelial neoplasia
COC	combined oral contraceptive
CPA	cyproterone acetate
CSM	Committee on Safety of Medicines (now Commission on Human Medicines)
DMPA	depot medroxyprogesterone acetate
DSG	desogestrel
DSP	drospirenone
EC	emergency contraception
ED	every day
EE	ethinylestradiol (oestrogen of the pill)
EHC	emergency hormonal contraception
EURUS	European Active Surveillance Study
FPA	Family Planning Association
FSH	follicle-stimulating hormone
GHG	greenhouse gas
GnRH	gonadotrophin-releasing hormone
GP	general practitioner
GSD	gestodene
GUM	genitourinary medicine
hCG	human chorionic gonadotrophin

HDL	high-density lipoprotein ('good' cholesterol)
HIV	human immunodeficiency virus
HPV	human papilloma virus
HRT	hormone replacement therapy
IUD	intrauterine device
IUS	intrauterine system
LAM	lactational amenorrhoea method
LDL	low-density lipoprotein ('bad' cholesterol)
LH	luteinizing hormone
LNG	levonorgestrel
LNG-IUS	levonorgestrel-releasing intrauterine system
NET	norethisterone
NFP	natural family planning
NGM	norgestimate
PCOS	polycystic ovary syndrome
PFI	pill-free interval
PIL	patient information leaflet
PMS	premenstrual syndrome
POP	progestogen-only pill
RCGP	Royal College of General Practitioners
SLE	systemic lupus erythematosus
SRE	sex and relationships education
STI	sexually transmitted infection
TOP	termination of pregnancy
TV	Trichomonas vaginitis
VTE	venous thromboembolism
WHO	World Health Organization
WTB	withdrawal bleeding

Evidence-base and competing interests

This book represents the personal opinions of John Guillebaud and Anne MacGregor, based wherever possible on published and sometimes unpublished evidence. When (as is not infrequent) no epidemiological or other direct evidence is available, clinical advice herein is always as practical and realistic as possible and based, pending more data, on the authors' judgement of other sources. These may include the opinions of Expert Committees and any existing Guidelines. In some instances the advice appearing in this book may nevertheless differ appreciably from the latter, for reasons usually given in the text and (since medical knowledge and practice are continually evolving) relates to the date of publication. Healthcare professionals must understand that they take ultimate responsibility for their patient and ensure that any clinical advice they use from this book is applicable to the specific circumstances that they encounter.

The authors have received payments for research projects, lectures, short-term consultancy work, and related expenses from the manufacturers of hormonal contraceptive products.

This book contains resource information but is not a substitute for more specific advice from your GP or family planning doctor, or the product information leaflets included in the pill packets. Virtually all information about the combined pill equally applies to the newer methods of combined hormonal contraception—the patch EVRA® and the vaginal ring NuvaRing®.

We have included information on the combined pill Yaz®. Although this pill is fully approved by the licensing authorities, at the time of publication the manufacturer had not yet announced when it will be marketed in the UK.

Part 1

Your choice of contraception

1

Why take the pill?

Jennie didn't bother with contraception as she'd heard that the pill was dangerous. Like many of her friends, she smoked. When one of her friends fell pregnant, Jennie realized she'd have to do something about contraception. She was surprised to find that, for her, the risks of smoking were much greater than taking the pill. She started on the pill, stopped smoking, and saved enough money for a long overdue holiday.

There are many myths and misconceptions about the pill, particularly about its safety. You can't lead your life without some risks, and when it comes to things like contraception, doing nothing can be risky too! So we've written this book to guide you through all the ins and outs of taking the pill. But, upfront, here are seven good reasons to choose the pill!

Because the pill is effective

The pill is as effective as any method currently available, short of sterilization. It is highly acceptable and unrelated to intercourse. It is almost 100 per cent reversible. However, these advantages are not unique, though, and apply also to injectables, implants, the intrauterine device (IUD), and the levonorgestrel intrauterine system (LNG-IUS).

Because the pill has beneficial effects

Improvement in symptoms of painful or heavy periods is something that is appreciated by nearly all pill users. There are also long-term benefits such as the lowered risk of cancer of the ovary, uterus, colon, and rectum. One way of looking at all of these benefits of the pill is as 'side-effects of *not* being on the pill'!

Figure 1.1 shows how frequent certain effects are, how the benefits match up against the unwanted effects, and by how much the pill increases or reduces their rate of occurrence.

Because the pill is reasonably safe—but some women are 'dangerous'

Risk factors multiply with each other and with the pill—but it is the woman with the risk factors, not the pill itself, that is largely responsible for the increased risk.

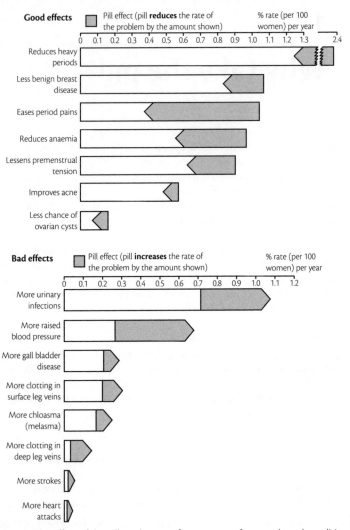

Figure 1.1 The effect of the pill on the rate of occurrence of some selected conditions (Royal College of General Practitioners' Study).
Note: all rates shown are the rates of attendance at the doctor's surgery and/or hospital admission for each condition.

And the opposite is also true: anyone without risk factors must have a much lower risk than average.

Consider this analogy. Insurance companies always require a high premium from students when they try to insure their cars; yet some of those students are very much safer drivers than the average (and may prove the fact in due course by having no accidents at all in the next 20 years). They always were safer drivers, but the risk estimates by the insurers had to be based on all kinds of students, including those who are irresponsible, who drive under the influence of drugs or alcohol, and so on.

Some risks are entirely in your own hands—like smoking, which is much more dangerous than taking the pill.

Because modern 'low-dose' pills are safer than older 'high-dose' pills

Earlier risk assessments were based mainly on research on higher-dose pills than are now in general use. When the pill was first available in the 1960s, each pill contained seven times the dose of oestrogen and 20 times the dose of progestogen used in current pills. So the early pills gave as much oestrogen in a day as is now taken in a week, and as much progestogen (norethisterone) as one current pill provides in a whole month!

Because serious side-effects are rare

If the frequency of a very rare event is increased several times, that is still a rare event. Fortunately, the serious conditions whose rate is increased by the pill, such as heart attacks and strokes, are extremely rare in women of child-bearing years. All the problems that are blamed on the pill also happen to women who have never had an artificial hormone in their lives and, as far as diseases of the circulation are concerned—which are among the most important risks—to men too.

Because pregnancy can be risky

When considering a balance of risk, we have to consider:

* The risk (if any) of the method itself.
* The risk of the pregnancies that will occur in a proportion of women due to failure of that method.

Pregnancy itself, whether its outcome is a baby or an abortion or a miscarriage, still carries some risks even in countries like Britain or the USA. Risks are far greater for women whose circumstances are different—especially in many developing countries where there is appalling, unacceptably high mortality through pregnancy, unsafe abortion, or labour without modern facilities. Worldwide, one woman dies that way each minute, nearly all in the less developed countries.

Because other things in life can be more risky

Even the highest estimates of risk due to the pill are of the same order as many other risks many of us take every year. Most of us are extremely vague and uninformed about the relative risks of daily activities. Figure 1.2 shows the time to reach a one in a million chance of death, which can be very short if you take up risky activities like motorcycling, or if you are over 35 and smoke. The longest time to reach that rate in the figure is for young non-smoking healthy pill takers.

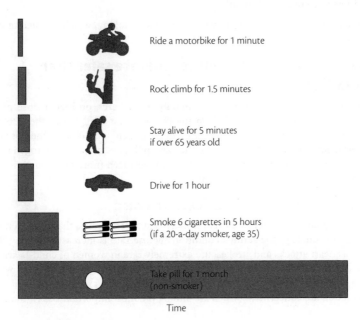

Ride a motorbike for 1 minute

Rock climb for 1.5 minutes

Stay alive for 5 minutes
if over 65 years old

Drive for 1 hour

Smoke 6 cigarettes in 5 hours
(if a 20-a-day smoker, age 35)

Take pill for 1 month
(non-smoker)

Time

Figure 1.2 Time required to have a one in a million risk of dying.
Data adapted from Minerva, *British Medical Journal* (1988) and from *Pharmacoepidemiology* (1994).

Unconvinced that the pill is right for you?

If you or your partner cannot feel confident about using the pill after discussing things with your doctor, or reading a book like this, then obviously you should avoid it. A doctor may perhaps insist there is no medical reason why you should not take it, but you should always have the final word.

2

What is the pill?

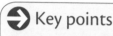 Key points

- The pill has been available since 1960.
- If taken correctly, it can be over 99 per cent effective at preventing pregnancy.
- It contains artificial oestrogen and progesterone, replacing the natural hormones produced by the ovaries.
- The pill hormones suppress the egg release from the ovaries each month, (ovulation), so pregnancy is prevented.

The 'pill' is a simple and very effective method of contraception taken by women to prevent unwanted pregnancies. It was first approved for use in the USA in 1960 and is now used by more that 100 million women worldwide.

The idea and the name of an oral contraceptive have been around for at least 2000 years. But nothing very useful came out of centuries of magic, mumbo-jumbo, and a great deal of trial and error. It was only when the normal processes of male and female reproduction were better understood that scientists could begin to devise more effective methods for blocking them. So in order to understand how the pill works, it helps to know first about the normal menstrual cycle.

The normal menstrual cycle

During their fertile years, women are unique in having a more or less regular monthly cycle of changes in their bodies. This cycle is caused by the ebb and flow in the bloodstream of various hormones or chemical messengers which are released into it by certain glands. The whole process is controlled by the brain, as is shown by the well-known fact that if a woman has a stressful emotional upset her periods can stop altogether for months at a time. The most important parts of the brain involved in the menstrual cycle are the hypothalamus and the pituitary gland (Fig. 2.1).

The pituitary gland is sometimes called the 'leader of the hormone orchestra' because it is so important. Yet it is really quite small, just the size of a large pea. The ovaries and uterus are also 'in the orchestra' and blood flows through them all, connecting the whole system together.

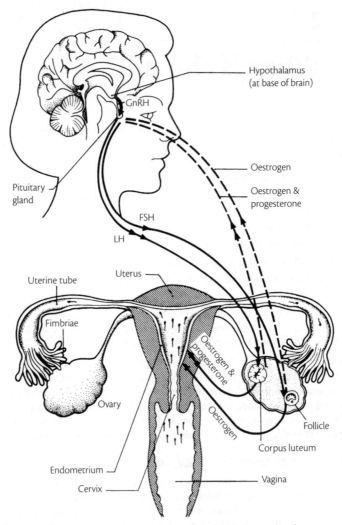

Figure 2.1 The female reproductive system: control of the menstrual cycle.

→ events of the first half of the cycle (follicular phase);

→→ the second half of the cycle (luteal phase);

– – – feedback effects (see pp. X–X);

FSH, follicle-stimulating hormone; GnRH, gonadotrophin-releasing hormone; LH, luteinizing hormone.

The menstrual cycle occurs because of a marvellously controlled interaction of hormones from the brain and the ovaries. The most important ones are two produced by the pituitary gland in the brain—follicle-stimulating hormone (FSH) and luteinizing hormone (LH)—and two from the ovaries—oestrogen and progesterone. These give their name to the first part of the menstrual cycle, the follicular phase, which starts from the first day of the menstrual period.

The follicular phase

Each cycle begins as a special hormone called gonadotrophin-releasing hormone (GnRH) is released from the hypothalamus. GnRH travels to the pituitary gland, stimulating the release of FSH. In turn, FSH travels in the blood to the ovaries.

The ovaries are about the same size as a peach-stone, though much less hard. Like the testicles of a man they have two functions: the production and the release of special sex cells (in this case eggs) and of hormones into the bloodstream. There are literally millions of potential egg cells in the ovaries of a baby girl before birth, but by the age of puberty the number has dropped to only 200 000—still more than enough for a lifetime. Normally only one egg is released from one or other ovary during each menstrual cycle, which commonly lasts for 28 days. Thus only about 13 are required each year. As no woman can be fertile for more than a maximum of about 40 years, only something over 500 eggs will ever be required. Occasionally, of course, more than one egg is released, leading, if pregnancy follows, to twins or perhaps triplets.

The immature eggs (oocytes) are contained in follicles. FSH from the pituitary stimulates about 20 or so follicles to grow each month. These maturing follicles manufacture oestrogen, which is released into the bloodstream.

Oestrogens are the fundamentally female hormones that influence the whole body, producing rounded contours, breast development, and many other features of femininity. They also stimulate the uterus to grow its new lining to replace the one that was shed at the previous menstrual period. Rising levels of oestrogen in the blood also have an important effect on the hypothalamus and the pituitary gland. This is known as 'negative feedback'.

What does 'negative feedback' mean?

- In general terms, negative feedback means that, if the level of a hormone in the blood goes *up*, the level of the stimulating hormone which caused it to go up is made to go *down*.

- In the menstrual cycle, this means for example: *up* ↑ oestrogen in blood causes *down* ↓ FSH.

- The opposite is also true: *down* ↓ oestrogen in blood causes *up* ↑ FSH.

As a result of negative feedback, the follicular phase rise in the level of oestrogen causes a fall in the pituitary gland's output of FSH.

Egg release from the ovaries

By about the 13th day of a standard 28-day cycle, the stimulated follicles have produced a rise of oestrogen in the blood to a peak level up to six times higher than it was on the first day. By negative feedback this has caused the level of the stimulating hormone FSH to drop. Now a most interesting and crucially different thing happens. Once the amount of oestrogen reaching the pituitary gland gets to a critical level, it releases into the bloodstream a sudden surge of LH. In other words, the *rise* in oestrogen is now causing a *rise* of a hormone from the pituitary. This is called 'positive feedback', to distinguish it from the negative type which operates all the rest of the time throughout the menstrual cycle.

While all this is happening, one particular follicle in one or other ovary will have grown and 'ripened' more than all the others. It is about 2 cm in diameter and looks like a balloon bulging the surface of the ovary. Its egg cell is also maturing, ready to be released and, should it get the chance, to be fertilized.

The surge of LH bursts the balloon, resulting in the release of a now mature and fertilizable egg (ovulation). If all goes well, this is picked up by the fimbriae of the uterine tube and transported towards the uterus (Fig. 2.2). As this occurs, some women notice pain in their lower abdomen, on one or other side, known by its German name Mittelschmerz.

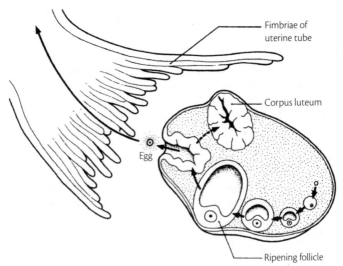

Fimbriae of uterine tube

Corpus luteum

Egg

Ripening follicle

Figure 2.2 Close-up of an ovary to show growth of follicles and formation of the corpus luteum after egg release.
Note: this is a sequence over 28 days, not a snapshot at any one time.

The luteal phase

During the second part of the menstrual cycle, which lasts on average 14 days, the particular empty follicle from which the egg came that month now produces the hormone progesterone, as well as oestrogen. It also turns yellow in colour, and so is given the name corpus luteum (which just means 'yellow body' in Latin). So this part of the cycle is called the luteal phase (Fig. 2.3a).

As oestrogen and progesterone are produced from the ovaries, they travel to the uterus. Their main business there is to thicken its lining with extra glandular tissue and blood vessels so that it is ready just in case a pregnancy starts that month.

Is the egg always released right in the middle of my cycle?

The time from egg release (ovulation) to the start of the next period is the only part of the cycle which is fixed in length, and lasts 14 (range 12–16) days. So if you have a period every 28 days, you would ovulate in the middle of your cycle. However, many quite normal cycles last less or more than the usual 28 days. If so, the variability is almost all in the time from the start of the period up to egg release. The first day of menstrual bleeding is always called day 1. So if, for example, a woman has a 35-day cycle, egg release would be expected on day (35 − 14 = 21).

Fertilization

If a woman has recently had unprotected sex, a sperm may reach the egg in the uterine tube and join up with it. This is fertilization. The fertilized egg starts just fourteen-hundredths of a millimetre in size. It begins to divide on its journey along the uterine tube towards the uterus, producing a fluid-filled sac (the blastocyst), which embeds itself in the prepared lining around the 19th day of the cycle. This is called implantation (Fig. 2.3b).

The embryo, as it becomes, now has just over a week to prevent the next period happening. This is vital otherwise it will be washed out by the menstrual flow. It does this by itself producing a special hormone, whose name is human chorionic gonadotrophin (hCG). This sends an urgent message in the bloodstream to the corpus luteum to make sure it keeps on producing oestrogen and progesterone, ensuring that the lining of the uterus is not shed and continues to provide nourishment for the developing embryo. These hormones also send messages to 'switch-off' the FSH and LH from the pituitary gland. This prevents further eggs being released while the woman is pregnant.

Menstruation: the period

If the egg is never fertilized or implantation fails (as it does about half the time), then the preparations for pregnancy come to nothing. The ovary stops producing

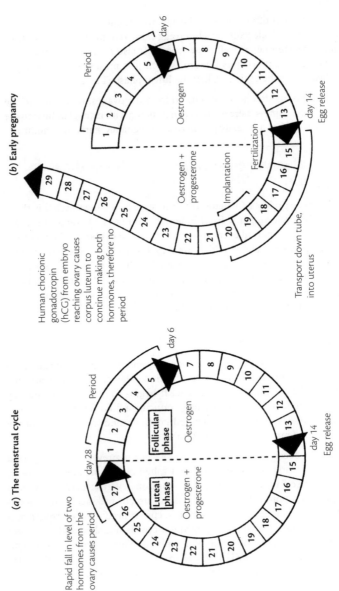

Figure 2.3 (a) The menstrual cycle; (b) early pregnancy.

Note: assumes standard 28-day cycle. Follicular phase is the part that varies, if the actual cycle is longer or shorter than 28 days.

oestrogen and progesterone at about 14 days after egg release as regularly as if it had a timing mechanism programmed to switch it off. This rapid loss of the hormones causes the lining of the uterus to break down and leave the body through the cervix and vagina. This causes the bleeding of the first day of the next period, which is day 1 of the *next* menstrual cycle.

All this may seem a detailed description but it is only a simplified version of what happens in a woman's body every month. 'Oestrogen' is in fact a family of hormones, of which the most important member in the menstrual cycle is oestradiol. Other hormones from the pituitary gland such as prolactin are involved; and the whole cycle can be affected by quite different hormones such as those from the thyroid gland, as well as by the nervous system.

How the pill was developed

Scientists in the early 1900s found that during pregnancy, the corpus luteum stops further egg release. In 1921, the Austrian Dr Haberlandt was the first person on record to suggest that extracts from the ovaries of pregnant animals might be used as oral contraceptives. But in the subsequent years many pharmaceutical companies feared the controversy that might result and were reluctant to apply these hormones (now synthesized) for contraception, though they were happy for them to be used in the treatment of various gynaecological conditions. In the early 1950s, Margaret Sanger, with her wealthy friend Catherine McCormack, provided the encouragement and resources to researchers that eventually led to the marketing of the pill. The leaders of this work were the chemists Russell Marker, George Rosenkranz, and Carl Djerassi, the biologists Gregory Pincus and Min Chueh Chang, and the obstetrician John Rock. They worked first with animals and then used a small group of human volunteers in Boston, Massachusetts. It soon became clear that the new hormones called progestogens, similar in structure to progesterone, were very effective contraceptives. Importantly, there were no immediate or obvious harmful effects.

Trials with a larger number of women began in Puerto Rico in 1956, supervised by a young gynaecologist called Celso Ramón-Garcia and Edris Rice-Wray (the first female physician involved in testing the pill). The trials were highly successful—until, that is, the chemists got rid of an impurity in the pills. This impurity was an oestrogen, mestranol. Immediately things began to go wrong. Irregular bleeding occurred and so did accidental pregnancies. So it was really by chance that the researchers learnt that a little oestrogen was necessary for maximum effectiveness and control of the cycle. When they put back in the amount previously present as an 'impurity', the combined pill was created. It took a few more years until June 1960 for the United States Food and Drug Administration to release the first combination oestrogen and progestogen birth control pill, Enovid-10.

The pill seemed to be safe but there was no certainty that it would prove to be so in the long term. So it was agreed from the start that these new and powerful medicines should be distributed only under close supervision, and the initial recommendation was that they should not be used for more than 2 years continuously. That idea, of using it only for a very few years at a time, to make sure it was fully reversible, has persisted in many people's thinking—despite the latest evidence which shows that ex-pill takers are *more* not less fertile than ex-users of alternative methods.

How the pill works

The combined oral contraceptive (COC) pill contains similar hormones to the oestrogen and progesterone produced by the ovary. Hence the pituitary gland is, as you might say, 'fooled' into thinking the woman is already pregnant. From its point of view, there is no need to send out hormones to stimulate the ovaries if there are already high levels of ovarian-type hormones. So the pituitary cuts drastically its output of the hormones FSH and LH. In particular there are no more of those mid-cycle 'surges' of a large amount of LH, which are essential for egg release. With so little of the hormones from the pituitary reaching them, the ovaries also go into a resting state, and produce minimal amounts of natural oestrogen and progesterone. Both the pituitary and the ovaries are like factories where the main production line has stopped, perhaps for a works' holiday, but small-scale production and essential maintenance are continuing. Such a factory can start full-scale production at short notice as soon as the workforce returns. Similarly, when a woman discontinues the pill, the hormone factories in the pituitary and ovaries rapidly return to normal working.

Figure 2.4 and Table 2.1 show the ways by which the usual combined pill and other combined hormone methods such as the patch and the ring operate to prevent pregnancy.

Table 2.1 How combined pills prevent pregnancy

1. Reduced FSH therefore follicles stopped from ripening and egg from maturing	++++
2. LH surge stopped so no egg release	++++
3. Cervical mucus changed into a barrier to sperm	+++
4. Lining of uterus made less suitable for implantation of an embryo (uncertainty, whether this effect is sufficient alone to stop a conception)	+
5. Uterine tubes perhaps affected so that they do not transport egg so well (uncertainty about this also)	+
Expected pregnancy rate per 100 women using the pill method for 1 year (compare use of 'No method' = 80–90)	<1–3

Note: the more plus signs the greater the effect

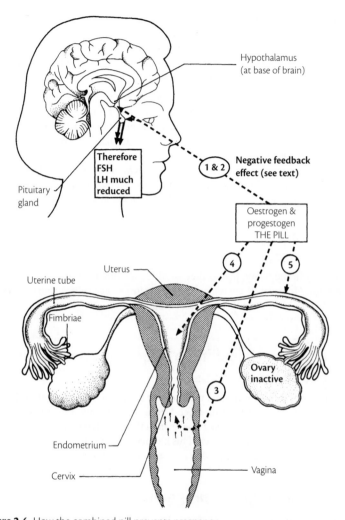

Figure 2.4 How the combined pill prevents pregnancy.

Note: numbers 1–5 are the contraceptive effects of the combined pill as shown in Table 2.1.

The main effect is to stop the normal hormone changes of the menstrual cycle and hence prevent both the maturing of follicles and actual ovulation—rows 1 and 2 in Table 2.1.

However, there is an important back-up mechanism to prevent conception even if egg release should occur. The most common reason for this 'breakthrough' egg release is forgetting to take tablets, especially after the pill-free time.

The slippery mucus which normally flows from the cervix in the fertile part of the cycle, and at that time is easily penetrated by sperm, is transformed by the hormones—actually the progestogen—into a scanty, thick material which produces a quite effective barrier to sperm. This third way by which the pill may work is still clearly preventing fertilization.

There are also changes in the lining of the uterus, which seem to make it less able to support and nourish a fertilized egg. But this fourth possible way is never needed by consistent pill takers—fertilization gets blocked first by one of the first three methods. In other words, even though it might theoretically be able to do so (and this is uncertain and disputed by some), the pill *never needs* to block the implanting of a very early pregnancy: a mechanism some people would call 'abortion' and would like to avoid. The fifth possibility, but unproven, is whether these hormones can be contraceptive through blocking egg transport.

If the pill stops release of eggs, what happens to the eggs?

They stay in the ovary, just as they would in a woman who was perpetually pregnant. However, there is always a steady loss of egg cells within the ovary, from before birth right through to the menopause.

Could using the pill for a long time affect when I get to the menopause?

Neither a combined hormonal method nor the progestogen-only pill (POP) (nor not ovulating for months on end because of having lots of babies and breastfeeding them all) seems to have any effect at all, whether to make the final period come later or earlier. This happens when your ovaries' supply of eggs runs out—something predetermined for each woman.

Effectiveness against pregnancy

When it is properly used, apart from the LNG-IUS (levonorgestrel-releasing intauterine system) and some injectables and implants, there is no more effective reversible method of family planning than the combined pill and its 'clones' such as patches and rings. This is explained because its back-up mucus method can work even if the prime effect of preventing release of an egg from the ovary were to fail. But failures do occur for two reasons: the method failing the user (which is rare) and the user failing the method (much move common, e.g. by forgetting some tablets). If this second cause of failure is added to the first, the total failure rate rises from less than one per 100 woman-years in consistent users to three, or even more in very erratic pill takers.

What does 'the pill has a failure rate of one per 100 woman-years' actually mean?

If 100 women used the pill for a year, one of them should expect to get pregnant. Put another way, if you the user were able to be fertile for 100 years, you would have an 'evens' chance of one pregnancy at the end of that time. For healthy women who take their pills absolutely regularly at the same time every day, the failure rate is reduced to as low as 0.3 per 100 woman-years with modern pills. This means just three pregnancies among 1000 users per year. But this is only with so-called 'perfect use': you need to realise that if you are a typical busy modern woman, it may be difficult to achieve this. Which is why some of the more forgettable alternatives in the next chapter are worth considering...

'Periods' and the combined pill

The pill hormones 'switch off' and replace the hormones produced during the natural menstrual cycle. Most pill-taking schemes are for 21 days followed by a 7-day break. The effect of stopping pill hormones during this break is to *imitate* the fall in the levels in the hormones that would otherwise happen at the end of a normal cycle. This causes shedding of the (rather thinner) lining of the uterus that the pill's hormones have produced during the previous 21 days—just like a period.

So if for some reason periods fail to happen while you are on the pill, it probably only means that there was too little artificially produced lining of the uterus that month for the stopping of the pill's hormones to lead to bleeding. 'Bad blood' is not 'piling up inside'. There just is *no blood to come away*. If you have been taking your pills regularly, the explanation is very unlikely to be pregnancy. Most importantly, *absence of hormone withdrawal bleeds is totally irrelevant to any risk to your future chances of having a baby*.

Some pill-takers notice the opposite—they bleed too often and on the 'wrong' (tablet-taking) days. This breakthrough bleeding (BTB) usually settles with time, provided that the pills continue to be taken correctly, but if it does not, this needs to be discussed with your pill provider.

How unnatural is the pill?

People are often concerned that it must be unnatural to suppress the normal cyclical activities of the ovary and of the pituitary gland. It can be argued that having menstrual cycles and periods is actually not entirely 'natural'. Biologically, suppression of the menstrual cycle for years at a time may in fact be a much more natural state of affairs. Before effective contraception became

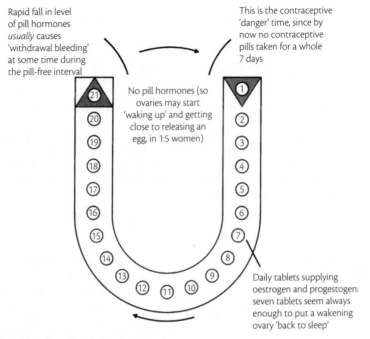

Rapid fall in level of pill hormones *usually* causes 'withdrawal bleeding' at some time during the pill-free interval

This is the contraceptive 'danger' time, since by now no contraceptive pills taken for a whole 7 days

No pill hormones (so ovaries may start 'waking up' and getting close to releasing an egg, in 1:5 women)

Daily tablets supplying oestrogen and progestogen: seven tablets seem always enough to put a wakening ovary 'back to sleep'

Figure 2.5 The pill cycle (21-day system).

Note: compare with Fig. 2.3a. The normal cycle shown there is taken right away and replaced by this simpler one. The bleeding from the uterus is caused just by withdrawal of the pill hormones. Pill taking is drawn in a horseshoe for the important reason that a horseshoe is a symmetrical object. Hence the pill-free interval can be lengthened, leading to the risk of conception, either side of the horseshoe: by forgetting (or vomiting) pills either at the beginning or at the end of the packet (see Chapter 13).

available, the normal thing was for a woman to be either pregnant or breast-feeding during all the childbearing years.

Although in many ways the effects of the pill are similar to those of pregnancy, they are by no means all the same: and pregnancy is anyway not free of risks. What is more, the hormones used are artificial rather than natural. The dosage of the two hormones is not exactly tailored to each individual. It is roughly constant for three weeks out of four rather than continuously varying as in the menstrual cycle.

So the most that can be said is that there are reasons to believe that the pill is *not nearly as 'unnatural'* as appears at first sight. What is puzzling is that some of the people who are worried by the so-called unnaturalness of the pill actually do something else which is even less 'natural' and certainly more dangerous—they smoke cigarettes!

3

What about other methods of contraception?

> ## ➔ Key points
>
> ◆ The pill is only one of a number of different methods of contraception.
>
> ◆ Each method has different advantages and disadvantages.
>
> ◆ Choice depends on how effective a method you need, your lifestyle, your health, and your sex life.
>
> ◆ Choice of method may change at different stages of life.

The wrong choice of contraception can lead to problems; not least an unwanted pregnancy, through using either an inefficient method, or a better method inefficiently. Although the pill is one of the most popular methods chosen, it is only one of a number of contraceptive options. Figure 3.1 shows, very approximately, some of the latest available information on current British usage of all the main methods of birth control. One conclusion must be that different couples make different choices: there is certainly no one ideal method.

Which method to choose

The final decision has to be your own: books and healthcare professionals can only answer your questions so far as the facts are known, and maybe give you some unbiased advice. But it is up to you to weigh up all the pros and cons, in consultation with your partner, and decide which method will suit you both best.

Your own 'best' method will depend on many things, among them: how crucial it is that you do not get pregnant; how much medical risk you feel prepared to accept; and how the actual method fits in with your sex life. Table 3.1 summarizes the most important pros and cons of the main recommended methods of contraception that are widely available. Methods with no user failures are the most effective as they don't rely on you remembering to use them!

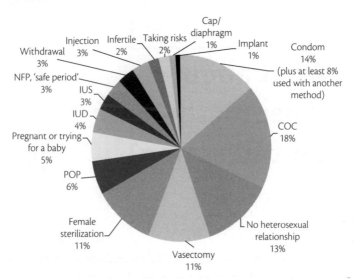

Figure 3.1 How birth control methods are used in the UK. Derived from the Omnibus Survey of the Office for National Statistics from a random probability sample of households surveyed in the year up to March 2007 (adjusted by the authors for respondents giving more than one answer).

Table 3.1 The main recommended and widely available methods of birth control

Reversible hormonal methods with no user failure	
Injectable (usually Depo-Provera®)	
Advantages	**Disadvantages**
• Pregnancy rate <1 per 100 woman-years	• Medical supervision required
• Each injection lasts for 12 weeks	• Irregular bleeding, but usually improves with time (or no bleeding, which can be an advantage)
• Independent of intercourse	
• Protects against pelvic infection and cancer of the uterus	
• Especially good for sickle cell anaemia	• Injection cannot be removed once given
• Oestrogen-free	• Delay in return of fertility, though no permanent fertility problems
• Not affected by any other medicines	• Minor problems such as weight gain and mood changes
	• Some of the possible long-term consequences unknown

Note: the user can make this fail but **only** by being late for the next injection.

Table 3.1 The main recommended and widely available methods of birth control (*continued*)

Contraceptive implants (Implanon®)

Advantages	Disadvantages
◆ Pregnancy rate <1 per 100 woman-years	◆ Medical supervision required
◆ Lasts 3 years	◆ Irregular bleeding
◆ Independent of intercourse	◆ Minor problems such as weight gain, breast tenderness, acne, and mood changes
◆ Protects against pelvic infection	
◆ Oestrogen-free	◆ Allergic skin reaction, rarely
◆ Rapidly reversible on rwwemoval	◆ Removal difficulties, rarely
	◆ Some of the possible long-term consequences unknown

The LNG-releasing IUS (Mirena®)

Advantages	Disadvantages
◆ Pregnancy rate <1 per 100 woman-years	◆ Medical supervision required
◆ Lasts for 5 years	◆ Insertion can cause discomfort
◆ Independent of intercourse	◆ Very slight chance of perforation of the wall of the womb
◆ Treats heavy and painful periods	
◆ Possible protection against pelvic infection	◆ Device may get expelled
◆ Oestrogen-free	◆ May cause prolonged spotting, especially in early months
◆ Local action so minimal side-effects	
◆ Rapidly reversible on removal	◆ May cause short-term medical side-effects, such as breast tenderness and acne

Reversible hormonal methods with user failure

Combined pill, patch, or ring

Advantages	Disadvantages
◆ Pregnancy rate <1 per 100 woman-years	◆ Medical supervision required
◆ Independent of intercourse	◆ Needs to be taken regularly (once-weekly patches may be easier for some women)
◆ Good cycle control and lighter 'periods'	
◆ Beneficial effects, especially on problems and diseases connected with the menstrual cycle, e.g. period pain, cancer of the ovary and uterus	◆ Minor side-effects common in first months of use
	◆ A slight chance of major problems such as thrombosis
◆ Choice of ways to use it (tablet, skin patch, or vaginal ring)	◆ Unsuitable for women with risk factors for thrombosis, e.g. heavy smokers over 35
	◆ Some of the possible long-term consequences are still unknown

(*continued*)

Table 3.1 The main recommended and widely available methods of birth control (*continued*)

The progestogen-only pill (POP)

Advantages	Disadvantages
◆ Pregnancy rate <1–4 per 100 woman-years (lower rate for Cerazette® and women over 45)	◆ Medical supervision required
	◆ Standard POP needs to be taken obsessionally regularly
◆ Independent of intercourse	◆ Minor problems, especially with irregular bleeding in the menstrual cycle
◆ Oestrogen-free	
◆ Can be used by smokers aged over 35 and others for whom the combined pill is not recommended, or is proving unsatisfactory	
◆ Good when breastfeeding, when it is nearly 100 per cent effective	

Reversible non-hormonal methods with no user failure
Copper intrauterine device (IUD)

Advantages	Disadvantages
◆ Pregnancy rate <1 per 100 woman-years	◆ Medical supervision required
◆ Lasts 5–10 years	◆ Insertion can cause discomfort
◆ Independent of intercourse	◆ Very slight chance of perforation of the wall of the womb
◆ Free of hormones	◆ Device may get expelled
◆ Effective for emergency contraception	◆ May cause period cramps, and heavy, prolonged, or unpredictable bleeding
◆ Rapidly reversible on removal	◆ Pelvic infection only a problem if lifestyle risks sexually transmitted infections (STIs)
	◆ Usually not first choice for women who have not yet had their family
	◆ Not as effective at preventing ectopic pregnancy (in the tubes)

Reversible non-hormonal methods with user failure
The male condom

Advantages	Disadvantages
◆ Pregnancy rate 2–15 per 100 woman-years; depends on careful use	◆ Needs very careful and consistent use
	◆ Forward planning necessary
◆ Widely available	◆ Not independent of intercourse
◆ Good for infrequent intercourse	

Table 3.1 The main recommended and widely available methods of birth control (*continued*)

Advantages	Disadvantages
◆ Lets a man take responsibility!	◆ Loss of sensitivity (much less with the newest designs)
◆ Visual proof that it has 'worked'	
◆ No medical risks	◆ Can slip off or rupture in use
◆ No medical supervision	◆ Latex ones may be damaged by oil-based chemicals
◆ Protects against STIs, including viruses such as those causing acquired immune deficiency syndrome (AIDS) (human immunodeficiency virus (HIV)) and cervical cancer (human papilloma virus (HPV))	
◆ Plastic versions (Durex Avanti® or Pasante Unique®) available if latex allergy	

The female condom (Femidom®)

Advantages	Disadvantages
◆ Pregnancy rate 5–15 per 100 woman-years	◆ Needs very careful and consistent use
◆ Visual proof that it has worked	◆ Forward planning necessary
◆ No medical risks	◆ Not independent of intercourse
◆ No medical supervision	◆ Particularly intrudes during foreplay
◆ Believed to protect against STIs	◆ Needs care to avoid the penis entering beside the outer ring, with complete loss of effectiveness
◆ Can be used before complete erection	
◆ Less likely to rupture than the male condom	
◆ During the penetrative phase, sensations of intercourse more normal (this noticed more by the male)	◆ Can become pushed in
	◆ Can be noisy (put on the music)!
◆ Not damaged by oil-based chemicals	◆ Relatively expensive

The cap plus spermicide (typically diaphragm)

Advantages	Disadvantages
◆ Pregnancy rate 4–8 per 100 woman-years with careful use, up to 10–15 otherwise	◆ Initial professional supervision required to size the cap and train in use
◆ More independent of intercourse than condoms—can be inserted in advance of intercourse	◆ Needs very careful and consistent use
	◆ Forward planning necessary
	◆ Seems a bit messy to some
◆ Neither partner usually notices any loss of sensitivity	◆ May increase the risk of bladder infections (less with other types of caps, e.g. Femcap®)

(*continued*)

Table 3.1 The main recommended and widely available methods of birth control (*continued*)

Advantages	Disadvantages
◆ If properly fitted and used, virtually no side-effects	
◆ Protects against some STIs and (very probably) cancer of the cervix	

Natural family planning (NFP), including Persona®

Advantages	Disadvantages
◆ Pregnancy rate 1–2 per 100 woman-years with careful use, otherwise 10–20 per 100 woman-years	◆ Very unforgiving of inconsistent use
◆ No side-effects	◆ Requires long durations of abstinence to be fully effective
◆ No hormones or other drugs, no devices, no procedures	◆ Except Persona®, NFP has to be learned from a trained teacher. It takes at least three cycles to learn
◆ Acceptable to all religions and cultures	◆ Events such as illness, stress, and travel may make some fertility indicators harder to interpret
◆ Empowers women, who feel more in tune with their body rhythms and sexuality	
◆ Actually benefits some couples' communication and relationships	
◆ Can be used to plan as well as avoid a pregnancy	

Methods which are not readily reversible

Sterilization in either sex

Advantages	Disadvantages
◆ Almost but not quite 100 per cent effective	◆ Not readily reversible—but pregnancy rates after reversal operations by experts can be better than 50 per cent
◆ Independent of intercourse	
◆ Nothing to be taken daily	◆ An operation is required with more or less discomfort and inconvenience
◆ Medical supervision and possible problems mainly during the year of operation	◆ Not 100 per cent, despite being so 'final'
◆ No known long-term medical effects of importance	◆ Late failures a long time afterwards can occur
	◆ Psychological effects of an irreversible method

Table 3.1 The main recommended and widely available methods of birth control (*continued*)

Female sterilization (blocking the uterine tubes)	
◆ Immediately effective	◆ Medical risks of the operation are greater than vasectomy, though still small
	◆ Usually requires admission to hospital and often (not always) a general anaesthetic
	◆ Less effective at preventing ectopic pregnancy

Male sterilization (vasectomy)	
◆ Almost completely safe medically	◆ Occasional short-term local complications of the operation, such as swellings or infection
◆ Can be done under local anaesthetic in about 10 minutes, as an out-patient, best by the no-scalpel technique	
	◆ Takes three or more months to be effective
◆ Easy to check effectiveness by doing sperm counts	◆ Some remotely possible, long-term effects still unknown, but available human evidence is very reassuring

Note: only condoms (male or female) realistically offer safer sex (protection against STIs, including HIV/AIDS). Even men who have had vasectomies must remember this!

Hormonal contraception

The COC pill and patch, and the POP are covered in great detail in the rest of this book. But even if you have already decided on the pill, it is still worth thinking about alternative options. In particular, three non-pill hormonal methods listed in Table 3.1 are worth considering.

Injectables

Depo-Provera® is the name for the progestogen injection of depot medroxy-progesterone acetate (DMPA for short), given in a dose of 150 mg into a muscle (usually the buttocks) once every 12 weeks. It is very effective since it mainly works by blocking ovulation, like the pill. Its failure rate is in practice lower even than the pill because there are no tablets to forget. It seems very safe medically, though no one can say it is risk-free.

◆ *Cancer*. World Health Organization (WHO) research has shown a strong protective effect against cancer of the lining of the uterus, and no proven increase in the risk of any other cancer.

◆ *Reversibility*. Research gives good evidence that there is complete return of fertility on stopping DMPA. Women take about 4 months longer after their first missed dose to conceive than after stopping other methods. Compared with ex-pill users, studies show that it takes women stopping the injection a bit longer to get pregnant in the first year. By the second year after stopping, the total number of conceptions is the same for both groups.

◆ *Other problems.* The main problems are excessive and irregular bleeding, often but not always going on to absent periods (which some people worry about but once they know it's harmless they realize it is a good side-effect!); and, in some women, weight gain, which can be very marked and unpredictable. Everyone should be forewarned about these side-effects, and also about the fact that DMPA cannot easily be removed if any side-effects do develop.

The possibility that DMPA may increase the risk of osteoporosis (thinning of the bones) through long-term lowering of blood oestrogen levels is still uncertain, and being studied. It is officially advised that this should be discussed with all users every 2 years, with the option to change to a different method if there is any concern. A few women at special risk of osteoporosis should not use DMPA (the main example being those with the eating disorder anorexia nervosa).

> Julie had several friends using DMPA, so she was keen to try this method. After her first injection, she started to feel more hungry, but remembered that the doctor had told her this could happen. She tried not to eat more than usual. She had no bleeding for the first 6 weeks and then started to get some spotting every day, which persisted until her next visit to the doctor. She had her second injection. By the time she returned for her third injection, the bleeding had settled and her appetite was back to normal. She was happy to continue with DMPA and enjoyed being period-free!

Contraceptive implants

Implanon® is the length of a matchstick but only 2 mm wide and is put just under the skin via a special needle under local anaesthesia (Fig. 3.2). Trained clinicians can insert this with minimum discomfort in about 1 minute, and remove it in 2 minutes. It works in a similar way to the pill, stopping ovulation, but is oestrogen-free. The main disadvantage is irregular bleeding. As with the injection and IUS, absent periods are an advantage!

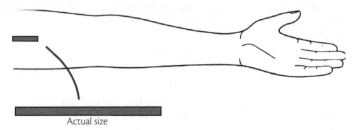

Actual size

Figure 3.2. Implanon® capsule implanted in the upper arm.

The levonorgestrel-releasing intrauterine system (LNG-IUS, or just IUS), marketed as Mirena®

As shown in Figure 3.3, the IUS is a T-shaped system releasing just 20 mcg per 24 hours of LNG from its special reservoir, through a rate-limiting membrane. This is sufficient for contraception over at least 5 years.

Its main contraceptive effects are local, by changes to the cervical mucus which block sperm and by suppressing the lining of the womb. This is why it also reduces bleeding and pain.

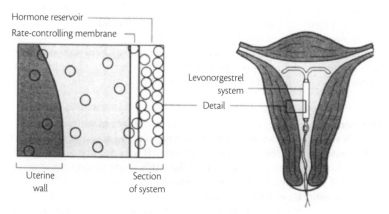

Figure 3.3. The LNG-IUS (Mirena®).

Users of this IUS can expect a dramatic reduction in amount and, after the first few months, in duration of their periods. Dysmenorrhoea (period pain) is also generally improved. Mirena® is the method of first choice for women with heavy periods and a tendency to get anaemia, who do not want the pill: a much easier option too than hysterectomy.

A common problem is the likelihood of bleeding in the first few months, which, although light, may be very frequent or continuous and can cause considerable inconvenience. Later on, amenorrhoea (absent periods) is a common advantage. It is well worth persevering, as the 'trickle' nearly always stops and then you either have light bleeds about once a month, or nothing at all!

Though this method is mainly local in its action, a small amount of hormone does get into the blood. So some women who are extra sensitive to hormones can still get hormonal side-effects such as acne and breast tenderness. If they happen at all, they usually improve over the first few months. The good news is that weight gain has not been shown to be a side-effect of the IUS.

Natural family planning (NFP)
Fertility-awareness methods

These are acceptable to the Roman Catholic Church and certain other religious groups who do not accept methods that are 'artificial'. This approach is also ideal for people 'spacing' their family (see Tables 3.1 and 3.2). For more details, including how you might visit a trained teacher in your local area to learn to use these methods well, visit http://www.fertilityuk.org.

Present methods depend mainly on combinations of calculations according to the length of previous menstrual cycles; on taking and charting the early morning temperature; and on learning to recognize certain changes in the cervical mucus, which usually occur before, during, and after the fertile time. If the woman cross-checks using more than one marker of ovulation, such as checking both mucus and temperature changes (the 'symptothermal' or multiple index approach), well-motivated women can control their fertility well.

Persona®

This personal contraceptive system measures changes in hormone levels in urine. It was first marketed in 1996 following years of research and is a very sophisticated micro-laboratory plus computer. It uses the first significant rise in natural oestrogen to show the start of the fertile phase (a red light comes on when a test stick dipped in urine is put into the hand-held electronic monitor). The green light comes back on when the LH surge (see Chapter 2) is detected by the system in the urine on the test stick and sufficient time is allowed thereafter for egg survival. Its internal computer is clever enough to keep updating and therefore individualizing the data on which it bases its decisions as to the start and end of the unsafe time. It is claimed that only 8 days' abstinence are usually required to achieve low pregnancy rates.

In the real world the manufacturer's claimed failure rate (six per 100 women or one in 17 in the first year of use) seems optimistic. Better results can be expected if unprotected intercourse is restricted only to the second 'green phase', after the egg is dead. But much worse failure rates are inevitable if a couple ever disobeys the red light. Although not cheap, many women find the price acceptable for a method completely free of health risk.

The lactational amenorrhoea method (LAM)

This is another very natural method that is not as widely publicized as it should be. It has a very acceptable success rate of 98 per cent, so long as all three questions can be answered 'No'—which means not relying on the method beyond 6 months after the birth. Thereafter a POP might be chosen, added to not so 'full' breastfeeding. Or, for even greater effectiveness, this could be your combination from early on, after the delivery.

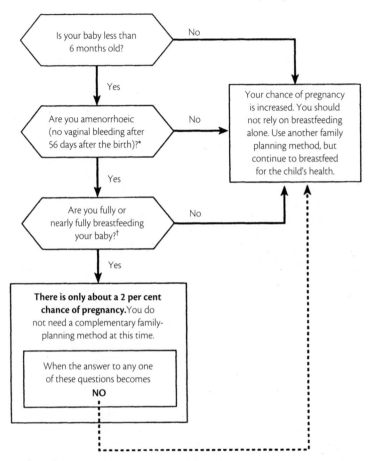

Contraception: your choices

Figure 3.4 The lactational amenorrhoea method (LAM).
Note: *Spotting that occurs during the first 56 days is not considered to be menstruation. †'Nearly' full breastfeeding means that the baby obtains almost 100 per cent of its nutrition from the mother alone, and certainly no solid food.

A lifetime of contraception

It has been calculated that a woman who wants just two babies will have to spend 86 per cent of her reproductive lifetime trying to avoid conceiving!

Some people will use only one or two methods of contraception throughout their lives; others will 'ring the changes' between the various methods. However, the choice of a method of contraception is a very individual thing and no one method is ever ideal and best for everyone, even within a particular age category.

Table 3.2 represents an ideal scheme and not all the satisfactory options are mentioned. It is assumed that the woman concerned will be a non-smoker and will, if she can, breastfeed her children. It is also assumed that she or her partner will use whatever method is chosen responsibly and consistently, and that they are fundamentally monogamous. Once a family is complete, sterilization of either partner can seem the ideal because it is so safe medically and so effective against unplanned 'afterthoughts'. Vasectomy is more effective and much easier to do. But reversible methods, such as banded copper IUDs and especially the Mirena® IUS, may be better choices. The IUS is ideal for many in the fifth, sixth, and seventh 'ages' of Table 3.2: by having one inserted a great many women whose periods have become either heavy or painful or both may be able to avoid having a hysterectomy (or even one of the less scary new techniques of uterine ablation which have been developed). It is also being increasingly used for a form of hormone replacement therapy (HRT), in combination with oestrogen by any chosen route.

Table 3.2 The 'seven' contraceptive ages of woman

Age	Suggested method
0 Birth to puberty	No method required. Responsible sex and relationships education (SRE) is essential, continuing through schooling
1 Puberty to marriage (or the equivalent)	Either (a) a barrier method, with emergency contraception back-up available; (b) the combined pill/patch/ring or Cerazette®/injectable/implant: outside of mutual monogamy always with a condom; or, if acceptable, (c) abstinence until the person's life-partner be found. The choice depends on factors such as religious views, perceived risk of STIs, and the frequency of partner changes and of intercourse
2 Marriage (or equivalent) to first child	First choice probably a pill, but could be one of various patches/rings/injectables/implants followed by a fertility-awareness method for some months before 'trying' for the first child
3 During breastfeeding	Either LAM, or POP, or any progestogen-only method, or a simple barrier method plus the breastfeeding. IUD or IUS, male or female injectable, or implant likely to be appropriate only if a longish gap is expected between pregnancies
4 Family spacing after breastfeeding	Continue with any method started during 'age' 3, or shift from an old-type POP to Cerazette®/combined pill/injectable/implant for greater effectiveness. Later, a banded copper IUD or IUS is progressively more appropriate, for a combination of the least long-term health hazards, efficacy, and reversibility

Table 3.2 The 'seven' contraceptive ages of woman (*continued*)

Age	Suggested method
5 After the (probable) last child	The first choice is an IUD or IUS, depending on whether periods are troublesome; other possibilities are any POP, or (if free of arterial or venous factors) a combined hormonal method, or injectable/implant according to choice
6 Family complete, family growing up	First choice still as '5': banded copper IUD, or the IUS if periods heavy or painful. According to choice, vasectomy would be generally preferable to female sterilization as it is more effective and easier to perform
7 Perimenopausal (not sterilized)	Contraceptive HRT, perhaps, such as the IUS plus oestrogen patch or implant. It is important to recognize that, at this age, a weaker contraceptive (e.g. foam or sponge) may be fully effective when combined with very reduced fertility

If you are a completely healthy, a non-smoker, with a normal body mass index (BMI), there is now also the definite option of staying on the combined pill right through to the menopause.

Whatever reversible method is used, it should not normally be abandoned until 1 year after the very last menstrual period (and then, if this was under age 50, 2 years is recommended). Pregnancy during this time is not entirely unknown following an unexpected delayed egg release!

Part 2

Keeping it safe

4

What causes the effects of the pill?

Key points

- The effects of the pill result from measurable changes in body chemistry.
- Many of these changes mimic pregnancy.
- Modern low-dose pills aim to have the minimum possible unwanted effects on the system.

All the good and bad effects must have their ultimate explanation in the chemistry of the body. More than 100 different laboratory tests on blood, urine, and other bodily fluids have given abnormal results in women on the pill (Table 4.1).

Many of the alterations are similar to those found in normal pregnancy. This is not surprising, as being on the pill in many ways mimics being pregnant. It is also somewhat reassuring. Pregnancy after all is a perfectly 'normal' condition, and many women have a whole succession of pregnancies and live long and healthy lives. On the other hand, pregnancy is linked with an increased risk of several conditions, including thrombosis, which we shall be considering shortly in connection with the pill.

In spite of much research, we have as yet no idea what some of the changes in body chemistry mean in practice. Quite a number, such as the oestrogen effects on blood-clotting factors, have an obvious link with known side-effects of the pill. Others, which may be responsible for known and unknown risks or benefits, remain as yet unexplained.

As a general working rule: *'if we can measure any substance in the pill user's body, we would like it to be normal—or as near normal as possible'.*

One consequence of the changes in the body chemistry is that whenever you visit a doctor it is most important to tell him or her that you are on the pill. This is particularly necessary if some specimen, such as a blood test, is going to be sent to a laboratory. The laboratory may be unable to interpret the results of the test satisfactorily unless this information is given.

Table 4.1 Some changes in body chemistry

	Blood level	Remarks
Liver		
Liver functioning generally	Altered in all users	These many changes cause no apparent harm to the liver itself, except in a tiny minority who develop jaundice. The liver is *involved*, however, in the production of most of the changes in blood level of substances shown in this table, including the important changes in blood sugar, fats, and clotting factors. These are minimal with the latest pills, but may partly explain the increased risk of thrombosis in arteries.
Albumin (the main protein of blood)	↓	
Transaminases (special liver enzymes)	↑	
Amino acids ('building blocks' for body protein)	Altered	
Blood sugar (glucose) after a meal	↑	
Blood fats (lipids)	Altered (mostly ↑)	
Clotting factors—generally	Mostly ↑	Both the pill and smoking affect these inter-related systems, connected with the risk of thrombosis. Fibrinolysis is enhanced in the blood, but *reduced* in the vessel walls.
Anti-thrombin proteins (special anti-clotting factors)	↓	
Fibrinolysis (the system to get rid of blood clots once formed)	↑	
Tendency for platelets to stick to each other (platelet aggregation)	↑	
Hormones		
Insulin	↑	These changes are thought to be connected with those affecting blood sugar and blood lipids (above).
Growth hormone	↑	
Steroid hormones from adrenal gland	↑	
Thyroid gland hormones	↑	
Luteinizing hormone (LH)	↓	Lowering the levels of these hormones is essential for the pill's contraceptive actions.
Follicle-stimulating hormone (FSH)	↓	
Natural oestrogen	↓	
Natural progesterone	↓	
Prolactin	↑	
Minerals and vitamins		
Iron	↑	This is a good effect
Copper	↑	Effects unknown, but not believed to cause any health risk in most pill users.
Zinc	↓	
Vitamins A, K	↑	
Riboflavin, folic acid	↓	
Vitamin B_6 (pyridoxine)	↓	
Vitamin B_{12} (cyanocobalamin)	↓	
Vitamin C (ascorbic acid)	↓	

(continued)

Table 4.1 Some changes in body chemistry (*continued*)

	Blood level	Remarks
Binding globulins	↑	These special substances carry hormones and minerals in the blood. Because their levels increase in parallel with them, the effective blood levels of the hormones and minerals are not much altered.
Blood viscosity	↑	
Body water	↑	This fluid retention explains some of the pill-related weight gain.
Factors affecting blood pressure	Altered	This is very complicated. Changes do not correlate as well as expected with the actual blood pressure levels.
Renin substrate	↑	
Renin activity	↑	
Angiotensin II	↑	
Immunity/allergy system		
Number of white blood cells	↓	
Immunoglobulins (antibodies) Function of the lymphocytes	Altered	

Note: in the table arrow up ↑ means the level usually goes up, arrow down ↓ means the level tends to go down. 'Altered' means that the changes are known to be more complex, with both increases and decreases occurring in different substances within the system concerned.

Effects on the blood levels of sugar and fats

The earlier pill types altered glucose or insulin levels and caused changes to lipids (blood fats), similar to those found in some women (and men) who have an above-average risk of heart attacks and strokes because of disease of their arteries. However, the newer pills in current use have fewer unwanted effects on the lipids and, with the exception of strokes, modern pills do not increase the risk of blood clots in the arteries unless you have an added risk factor such as smoking.

Effects on blood levels of minerals and vitamins

The vitamin and mineral changes have not been shown to cause any harm at all to most women. *So pill users should not feel pressurized to take extra vitamins*, whether by an expensive 'pill protection formula' or from any other source. The main thing is to rely on a normal diet, including plenty of fruit and vegetables.

Folic acid and vitamin B_{12} help to produce normal red blood cells. Anaemia due to the shortage of either of these substances has only been described (and very rarely) in pill users on poor diets. The more frequent kind of anaemia—due to shortage of iron—often improves on the pill.

Fluid retention and weight gain

Fluid retention occurs more in some women than others, and is due to some complicated adjustments to body chemistry among pill users. Except in certain types of heart and kidney disease, this seems to be quite harmless. It does, however, cause some of the weight gain for which the pill is often blamed, perhaps about a kilogram or so, just because of extra water being in the body. This is very temporary and the weight is lost if the pill is stopped.

Fear of gaining weight is one of the things that most puts women off the pill. Yet in a study of two modern ultra-low-dose pills (Femodette® and Mercilon®), 70 per cent of the users of both brands stayed the same weight in the first year (plus or minus 2 kg). The remaining 30 per cent was split exactly—half of the women lost more than 2 kg and the other half gained more than 2 kg. That really adds up to the pill having had a zero effect with random or unconnected ups and downs over the year. But you can clearly see how the 15 per cent of women who put on the weight would be bound to blame the pill, quite unfairly.

Some users notice in fact that they shed the extra weight regularly during the 7-day break from pill taking each month. Yasmin® and Yaz® can help a few women who get symptoms such as breast swelling and bloatedness along with this kind of cyclical fluid retention. They contain the progestogen drospirenone, which is a weak diuretic, helping to get rid of fluid from the body.

If, despite all that, weight gain after going on the pill seems to be a real problem, consider trying a different brand before you throw your packets away, or fix up a different method of contraception—pregnancy causes weight gain too!

Immunity and allergy

Several studies have all showed that pill users are more likely than non-users to have various infections, including chickenpox, gastric flu, and respiratory and urinary infections. Other inflammations, of soft tissues or of the bowel (tenosynovitis, bursitis, synovitis, and Crohn's disease), have also been reported more commonly in pill users.

These facts suggest but don't prove that the pill can alter immunity. In addition, various skin troubles are often connected with allergy, and eczema, for instance, was twice as common in pill users in one study. Women can also develop an allergy to either the progestogen or the oestrogen of the pill itself. This occurs even more rarely than with other commonly used drugs such as penicillins, but can show itself by troublesome rashes or by painful swollen joints (polyarthritis). These clear up completely only when the pill is stopped, and would recur if the same hormone were to be given again. Whether allergies to other substances happen more readily because the pill is being taken is not so clear, though the reported increased rate of hay fever is suggestive.

Another possibility is an allergy to a person's own tissues causing so-called autoimmune diseases. It does appear that the pill can sometimes aggravate the symptoms and signs of one of these, systemic lupus erythematosus (SLE), which affects connective tissues in the body. The immune/allergy system is involved in causing several types of thyroid disease and arthritis. As the pill seems to have protective effects on some of these (e.g. rheumatoid arthritis), perhaps some good effects too are due to an alteration in this system.

5

What are the benefits?

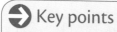 **Key points**

- The pill is nearly 100 per cent effective at preventing pregnancy.
- The pill does not interfere with intercourse.
- The pill is nearly 100 per cent reversible.
- The pill has a number of non-contraceptive benefits.

The contraceptive benefits of the pill are obvious. But many of its benefits have nothing to do with contraception (Table 5.1). All the other good effects can have considerable advantages for some women—indeed, they may choose to take the pill even if they don't need it for contraception.

The breasts

Benign breast disease (BBD)

BBD is the general term used to include a number of non-malignant problems of the breast, which may be called fibromas, 'fibrocystic disease', and a variety of other names. They all refer to more or less generalized lumpiness of the breast. Here is a definite plus point for the pill, as the usual type of this breast trouble tends to be less common during pill use, especially long-term pill use. However, the paradox is that BBD is a 'risk factor' for breast cancer. So, although the pill reduces the risk of getting BBD in the first place, doctors exercise extra caution if the breasts have the problem already, especially if a lump has had to be operated on. Established BBD is now seen as a so-called 'relative contraindication' to using the pill.

Breast tenderness

Tenderness can be part of the whole range of symptoms of premenstrual tension, or it can occur alone. In some unfortunate women the tenderness can be so extreme that for a few days before each period they cannot bear their breasts being touched, even by clothing. If you have this problem (even if not quite as bad as that), you may find you are better off while on the pill. A few women actually report breast tenderness for the first time on the pill or patch, especially during the early months. Breast tenderness and discomfort on one brand may often be helped by switching to a less oestrogen-dominant one.

Table 5.1 Non-contraceptive effects of the combined pill

Good effects	
Common	**Uncommon or rare**
◆ Benign breast disease—less	◆ Bones—prevents osteoporosis
◆ Breast tenderness—usually less	◆ Cancer of the ovary—less
◆ Menstrual cycle improved:	◆ Cancer of the endometrium—less
· More regular bleeding	◆ Cancer of the rectum and of the colon—less
· Timing of one's 'periods' can be controlled	◆ Duodenal ulcers—?less
· No ovulation pain	◆ Ectopic pregnancies—much less
· (Less premenstrual tension)	◆ Endometriosis—less
· Less period pain	◆ Fibroids—fewer troubles
· Less heavy bleeding, therefore:	◆ Ovarian cysts—less
· Less anaemia	◆ Rheumatoid arthritis—less
◆ Pelvic infection—less	◆ Thyroid disease—?less
◆ Poisoning—almost impossible	◆ Toxic shock—?less
◆ Skin improvements	
· (Acne—less with some pills)	
· (Unwanted hair growth—less with some pills)	
◆ Trichomonas vaginalis—?less	
◆ Wax in the ears—less, overall	

Note: brackets on their own mean the pill can have real but quite opposite effects in different women, e.g. some pill takers report increased premenstrual tension.

The reproductive system
The menstrual cycle and periods

Many women have period problems including short cycles (every 3 weeks or so), irregular periods, ovulation pain, premenstrual tension, painful periods (dysmenorrhoea), and heavy periods leading sometimes to anaemia. For most women, almost every period problem is improved if they take the pill. This is because the pill abolishes the natural menstrual cycle altogether, and replaces it with a cycle caused by stopping the hormones for 7 days in each 28. See Box 5.1.

Ectopic pregnancy

This is the name for a pregnancy in the wrong place—usually in a tube, instead of in the cavity of the uterus. It can lead to dangerous internal bleeding. While a woman takes the pill, she is (almost) completely protected from this, because

Box 5.1 Periods and the pill

- *Regular:* your 'periods' can be accurately predicted.

- *Lighter:* you are much *less likely to become anaemic*. This is because pill users tend to have lighter periods and therefore to lose less iron from the body each month.

- *Less period pain:* period pains are caused by excessive contractions of the uterus, due mainly to pain-producing substances called prostaglandins. The thinner type of womb lining that develops in women on the pill causes less prostaglandins to be released.

- *No ovulation pain:* Mittelschmerz means 'middle pain' and refers to the pain which signals ovulation or egg release. Quite a lot of women feel this slight ache in the groin on one or other side around the middle of the cycle, which in some months can be quite severe. This pain is due to the growing follicle stretching the ovary, before it ruptures to release the egg. When this happens, there may also be a small amount of painful internal bleeding. Because the pill prevents ovulation, this pain is stopped.

- *Less premenstrual syndrome (PMS):* many sufferers from premenstrual symptoms of depression, irritability, feelings of bloatedness, weight gain, tenderness of the breasts, backache, and headache find these improve if they take the pill—especially if they tricycle it or take it continuously

- *Ability to control the periods:* if you have a special event such as a holiday or exams, you can run two packs together to skip a period. You can also as a 'one-off' ploy start a new pack early, with a shorter pill-free week, to make sure you never have periods at weekends. It is even possible, though not yet the normal routine, to take the combined pill continuously 365/365 (Chapter 12) and (often) have no vaginal bleeding at all.

she is not releasing eggs. Damaged tubes are the main cause of the problem, so if she has these she could still get an ectopic pregnancy later, after stopping the pill. But the pill makes even this less likely because it reduces the risk of pelvic infection while it is taken and, worldwide, that is the main cause of tubal damage.

Endometriosis

Endometriosis is an uncommon condition that is not entirely understood but causes misery to some women. Each month they suffer from a severe aching or bruising pain before and during the period, worsened by intercourse. Endometriosis is due to the same kind of tissue that normally lines the uterus being present in the wrong place—such as in the ovaries (where it is one cause of cysts) or elsewhere in the reproductive system, or even further afield.

How this tissue reached these sites is often unexplained. But, just as it bleeds in its correct place, in the uterus, so this wrongly situated endometrium bleeds regularly at period times; and bleeding into the tissues without being able to escape, like womb-bleeding can, causes bruising pain. Abolishing periods by taking the pill continuously or tricycling with a high-progestogen combined pill is often used to prevent relapse of endometriosis.

Fibroids

Fibroids are lumps of muscle and fibrous tissue, which can grow on the uterus. They are not cancerous. They are so common that most women get them eventually, though the size can vary from a pinhead to (rarely) something as large as a melon. Most women don't need treatment for fibroids. However, they are one of the causes of excessively heavy periods (menorrhagia) in some women in their late thirties or forties. In the past, the treatment was often with a hysterectomy (removal of the uterus).

Research shows that fibroids are *less* commonly diagnosed in users of the pill than in non-users, and if they are present are *less* likely to require hospital referral. The heavy periods which lead to the diagnosis of fibroids if they are present simply do not happen on the pill, because the pill almost always diminishes bleeding from the uterus.

If fibroids are diagnosed, one of the more progestogen-dominant brands is best or a progestogen-only method, such as Depo-Provera® or the IUS. In most women the pill reduces the bleeding trouble that they may cause but in a few individuals the fibroids may enlarge. If you have fibroids, you may be advised to have regular annual examinations, with ultrasound scans as required.

Ovarian cysts

Certain ovarian cysts known as functional cysts are less common in women on the combined pill. These are not tumours: they are balloons containing fluid entirely surrounded by a tissue capsule, developing within the ovary. They are thought to arise because of minor imbalances in the normal menstrual cycle. They start life as a follicle, stimulated to grow by FSH during the first half of the cycle, as described in Chapter 2. However, instead of the follicle rupturing to release an egg, or simply losing its fluid and virtually disappearing like the other 19 or so stimulated follicles do, the mechanism can go a bit wrong and a particular follicle goes on accumulating fluid to produce a cyst. This can be just a few centimetres in size or grow to a fluid-filled bag up to 10 cm or more in size.

Such cysts are usually painless but can sometimes cause quite bad pain, including pain on intercourse. They may cure themselves (by losing their contained fluid), or rarely lead to an emergency laparoscopy operation—especially if the cyst causes the whole ovary on either side to twist (torsion).

The good news for pill takers is that the ovaries are made inactive and no follicles are stimulated to accumulate fluid ready for ovulation or to make a cyst. There is a suspicion that the very lowest-dose pills may not suppress the activity of follicles so well and so may produce less of this benefit. The POP actually increases the risk of these functional cysts.

Polycystic ovary syndrome (PCOS)

This is a different kind of cyst-producing condition in which little cysts appear all around the outside of the ovaries. It produces the wrong balance of hormones, including more androgen (male hormone) than would be normal in a woman (of course some is produced by all women). This excess androgen causes acne and abnormal hair growth (hursutism) and the periods become very irregular or non-existent. It is diagnosed by an ultrasound scan of the ovaries. The pill can be very beneficial in the treatment of symptoms of PCOS —so long as the right kind of pill, an oestrogen-dominant one, is chosen. We now have three whose progestogen is *anti-androgenic* (Yasmin®, Yaz®, and Dianette®) which are often best for treating PCOS—while still being contraceptive.

Pelvic infection

Pelvic infection is usually due to an STI, particularly chlamydia but also gonorrhoea. It can seriously damage the uterine tubes, leading to infertility and/or the risk of ectopic pregnancy. Researchers have found that pill users have half the rate of this kind of infection, compared with those using no contraception. This good effect is probably due mainly to the same mucus changes in the cervix caused by progestogen. The altered mucus seems to obstruct bacteria as well as sperm. This reduces, but does not of course remove, the risk of pelvic infections spreading up to the tubes. It is a useful benefit but not something to rely on—more effective choices to avoid these STIs are monogamy or condoms.

Toxic-shock syndrome

The toxin (poison) is produced by the *Staphylococcus* bacterium, which multiplies in the vagina. As the toxin reaches the bloodstream, it causes a high fever, bright red skin rash, vomiting, diarrhoea, and low blood pressure. The condition was given much publicity because of its link with menstrual tampons. It is extremely rare, the more so if women change their tampons frequently. But it is dangerous, and evidence is emerging that pill users are even *less* likely to get it than other women.

Trichomonas vaginitis (TV)

There is some evidence from studies that this common STI, causing an itchy, fluid vaginal discharge, is *less* frequent than usual among pill users. However, there is no proof as yet of this beneficial effect. If it occurs, as when chlamydia is diagnosed, it is vital that you and your partner(s) are properly treated at a genitourinary medicine (GUM) clinic.

The digestive system
Duodenal ulcers

Research shows that women on the pill are less likely than non-users to require treatment for severe indigestion due to this type of ulcer. However, it is hard to rule out the possibility that an anxious person who is prone to such ulcers will also be unlikely to use the pill.

Bones and joints
Arthritis

Women on the pill are less likely to suffer from the more severe forms of the very troublesome joint disease known as rheumatoid arthritis. Though some studies have not shown this good effect, most experts now think that use of the pill is definitely beneficial.

Osteoporosis

Osteoporosis means thinning of the bones, making them more likely to fracture even without much trauma. Although fractures mainly affect women past the menopause, osteoporosis often begins earlier, as the ovaries work less well in the years leading up to the final menstrual period. Unless they are treated with oestrogen, younger women who are short of oestrogen from their own ovaries due to amenorrhoea—often connected with anorexia and weight loss, and sometimes in athletes—can also be affected.

If due to lack of oestrogen, osteoporosis can be prevented by the pill, as by HRT. As a result, pill takers have been found to reach the menopause with better bone density than other women.

So the pill can be of real value to older women free of risk factors who also want contraception.

Jilly is 44 and, apart from a 4-year break to have her two children, she has taken the pill since she was 20. She is healthy, not overweight, and does not smoke but is worried that she is going to follow in her mother's footsteps with a troublesome menopause and osteoporosis. When she stopped the pill, she noticed that she became very irritable before her periods, which were painful and heavy. Back on the pill, these problems have disappeared and she is delighted that the pill can help prevent her from suffering the same problems as her mother.

The skin

Acne

Acne occurs chiefly because the tiny ducts or passages leading from the grease-producing glands of the skin, especially in the face and on the back, tend to get blocked. The oestrogen in the pill may help to stop this happening. This improvement is more likely with an oestrogen-dominant brand using one of the new progestogens, such as Marvelon®, Cilest®, Yasmin®, Yaz®, or, in some cases, Dianette®. There are also other treatments that a family doctor might use, including tetracycline antibiotics and retinoids, which must be used together with effective contraception. Referral to a dermatologist may be necessary in the worse cases or those with hirsutism as well. Women with moderately severe acne or unwanted hair very often have PCOS (see above), so you might consider asking if an ultrasound scan should be done.

Increase in facial or body hair (hirsutism)

Hirsutism is fortunately very rare with the modern low-dose pills, and nearly always has another cause (i.e. being on the pill is a coincidence). Normally it's the other way around—an oestrogen-dominant pill with one of the new progestogens such as Yasmin®, Yaz®, or Dianette® may help in the treatment of this. Extra hair may also have to be removed with the help of electrolysis or similar treatment from a skin specialist.

Less greasy hair and less wax in the ears

The wax-producing glands of the ears are affected in the same way by the hormones of the pill as the grease-producing glands of the skin and hair. Studies show that women on the pill (primarily the oestrogen-dominant ones) are less likely to have their ears syringed for wax.

Toxicity (poisoning)

One of the very good points about the pill is that it seems to be almost impossible to take a fatal or even dangerous overdose. Toddlers have been known to swallow dozens of their mother's pills and, apart from feeling or being rather sick, have ended up none the worse for the experience. If the patient should be a baby girl, she may well have a 'period', because the hormones have stimulated the lining of her tiny uterus. Hence, as her body gets rid of the swallowed hormones, a harmless withdrawal bleed follows in the usual way. However, this does not stop the need for all medicines to be kept secure and out of the reach of children!

6

What are the unwanted side-effects?

 Key points

- Different women react to different pills in different ways.
- Most side-effects are apparent when first starting the pill and usually resolve with continued use.

Although the pill suits the majority of women, it is not good news for everybody—unwanted effects such as those listed in Table 6.1 can occur. Most are a nuisance, not dangerous. Thrombosis, heart attacks, strokes, and cancers are discussed in detail in Chapters 7 and 8. See Chapter 15 for management of side-effects.

The reproductive system
Bleeding disturbances

BTB is 'spotting' or sometimes a heavier blood loss, coming on at any time during pill taking. It happens for the same reason as the normal pill 'period': too little of the pill's hormones reaching the lining of the uterus. Similarly, a woman can have no bleeding during the pill-free week. Provided pregnancy is excluded, this can be an advantage.

Fertility
Return of fertility after stopping the pill

Doctors have always been aware of the possibility that because the pill acts by switching off the normal menstrual cycle, it might affect fertility when the pill is stopped. In fact, the results of research studies are very reassuring that the pill does not cause infertility. One recent study found that if women had used the pill for 5 years or more before they stopped to try for a baby, they conceived faster than women who had never taken the pill!

Table 6.1 Effects of the combined pill

Bad effects	
Common	**Uncommon or rare**
◆ Absent bleeding in pill-free week	◆ Breast pain
◆ (Allergies)	◆ Cancer of the breast—uncertain
◆ Bleeding on pill-taking days	◆ Cancer of the cervix
◆ Breast enlargement	◆ Chloasma or other skin troubles
◆ Cramps and pains in legs, or in arms	◆ Contact-lens troubles
◆ Cystitis and other urinary infections	◆ Delayed return of fertility
◆ (Depression)	◆ Fibroids
◆ Ectopy of the cervix with increased vaginal discharge	◆ Gallstones
◆ Fluid retention/bloatedness	◆ Heart attacks
◆ Gum inflammation	◆ Hypertension
◆ Headaches	◆ Jaundice
◆ (Loss of libido)	◆ Milky fluid from breasts
◆ Migraine	◆ Phlebitis—thrombosis of superficial veins
◆ Nausea	◆ Strokes
◆ Reduced resistance to some infections	◆ Tumours of the liver—adenoma and very rare primary cancer
◆ Weight gain	◆ Venous thrombosis with or without pulmonary embolism

Note: brackets mean that the pill can have opposite effects in different women, e.g. some pill takers report increased libido; allergies can improve or worsen.

Fertility goes down with age. So sometimes the problem is partly connected with delaying too long before trying for a baby. This is a most important point. All methods of contraception share a common 'side-effect': they give modern women the freedom to delay starting their family, but this can sometimes mean they let their 'biological clock' tick for a bit too long. This is how some women suffer from infertility at 35, yet could have conceived easily at 20.

> ## We have been trying to have a baby since stopping the pill (or ring or patch) with no success yet. Was it to blame and should we have tests done?
>
> Between 10 and 15 per cent of all couples are not pregnant after 'trying' for a whole year. So it *could* be a coincidence, especially if you're a bit older now (since not starting to try till above age 35 tends to mean taking longer). Discuss referral for tests with your doctor if you have been without periods for 6 months or more, but if:
>
> ◆ the periods have returned *and*
>
> ◆ *you have no bad pain symptoms* (which could be due to endometriosis) and
>
> ◆ you are under 30
>
> then it is usually fine to keep trying for up to a year before being investigated for a possible fertility problem.

Very few women, perhaps one in 200 who stop the pill, develop amenorrhoea—absence of ovulation and periods—for over 6 months. This is not normal and should be investigated. Experts believe that in only a few—if any—such cases was the pill truly connected and, even then, only by bringing out a natural tendency. Reassuringly, it is also now possible to treat this fertility problem when there are no periods with almost 100 per cent success.

Effect of the pill on a pregnancy

Providing the pill is discontinued well before conceiving, researchers have failed to detect any consistent increase—or decrease—in any type of abnormality. So, any woman who conceives less than 3 months after stopping the pill should not be concerned. Like all women planning a pregnancy, you should take 0.4 mg of folic acid daily, which you can buy from any chemist. This should be taken *before* conception and for the first 12 weeks of pregnancy. A good diet throughout pregnancy, as well as steering clear of all avoidable chemicals (certainly cigarettes and alcohol), is important.

If you had been taking the pill before realizing you were pregnant, it is highly unlikely that the pill will cause any problems. The rate of birth defects in studies of women who took the pill when pregnant is no higher than would be expected in any group of women having a planned baby. So, if your baby is born with a serious defect, it is unlikely to have been caused by the pill—not many people realize that 20 in 1000 of *all* babies have a serious defect at birth.

The breasts
Breast enlargement

Most users of the pill notice some enlargement. The increase, not normally more than one bra-cup size, is mainly fluid building up through the pill cycle, and it often lessens in the pill-free time. It tends to reach its maximum by the second packet of pills, and in the absence of weight increase your bra size is then likely to be stable until you come off the pill method again.

Milky fluid from the nipples

Prolactin produced by the pituitary gland is a hormone whose levels in the blood tend to go up in pill takers, and in a few this leads to a milky fluid coming from the nipples. This can be a nuisance and should always be mentioned to your doctor. The level of the hormone should be measured, as, if it is particularly high, it could perhaps be coming from a pituitary adenoma, or micro-adenomas, which need specific medical treatment. Although the pill does not cause adenomas, it should usually be discontinued during treatment.

Breastfeeding

The combined pill can affect the volume and quality of milk flow in women who are breastfeeding after recently having had a baby, so is best not used. In contrast, the POP does not interfere with the milk and, in combination with full breastfeeding, is close to 100 per cent effective at preventing pregnancy.

The brain and central nervous system
Depression

The link between depression and the pill is a bit complicated. Firstly, the pill most commonly improves the kind of depression some women get premenstrually in the normal menstrual cycle. Secondly, research shows that the pill does not increase the risk of severe depression—or indeed of any mental disorder so bad as to require a specialist opinion or admission to hospital. Despite this, depression is one of the most common reasons women give for stopping the pill. In addition, most doctors have seen mood improve in some women when they stop taking the pill, and worsen whenever they start it again.

Migraine

Migraine is episodic attacks of moderate-to-severe headaches, which are disabling and are accompanied by sensitivity to light and sound, and feeling sick or even vomiting. They are often, but not invariably, one-sided. There is no concern about using the pill if you have this type of migraine *without* aura. Indeed, many women taking the pill notice an improvement in their migraine. In contrast, migraine *with* aura, in which very specific disturbances of vision occur *before* the headache, can start for the first time in pill users. Because it has been linked to increased risk of stroke, women with this type of migraine should not use the pill (see Chapter 9).

Non-migraine headaches

Research has shown that headaches can be more common in the first few months of taking the pill, but usually settle with time. So unless they are particularly troublesome, it is worth persevering with the pill. Apart from taking painkillers if necessary, use the very lowest-dose pill that suits you in other ways. If they mainly or only come in the pill-free time, you could ask about reducing the number of pill-free breaks a year by tricycling or taking the pill continuously, 365/365 (Chapter 12).

The eyes

Contact lenses

Very occasionally, contact-lens users find that their eyes get sore for the first time when they start the pill. A possible reason seems to be that there is a slight corneal oedema, or increase in the amount of fluid in the cornea (the transparent covering in front of the iris). Make sure you give the eyes a rest from lens wearing where possible and discuss the matter with your optician.

The digestive system

Nausea (queasiness)

With modern pills nausea is uncommon, except in underweight women. It can be particularly bad during the first few days of pill taking after the pill-free time for the first two or three cycles and then usually disappears for ever.

The liver and gall bladder

The liver has special receptors for sex hormones, so the pill can influence its many functions (see Chapter 4). The alterations—in clotting factors and blood fats, for example—mean that the liver is often behind most of the unwanted effects of the pill even if they occur elsewhere in the body.

Jaundice

Jaundice is the sign of several liver diseases that make the skin and the eyeballs go a yellow colour. The reason for this is an increase in the amount of a yellow substance called bilirubin in the blood. If the liver is damaged from any disease causing jaundice, the pill is stopped until after recovery.

Gallstones

The gall bladder is the reservoir for bile. Bile is a very saturated solution, and it has been shown that the hormones of the pill tend to make it even more saturated. In a few women this can lead to gallstones forming.

The urinary system

Cystitis and other urinary infections

Cystitis is the name for infection of the bladder caused by bacteria in the urine. This usually needs treating with an antibiotic. Even when there are no symptoms, bacteria are grown more commonly from the urine of pill users than other women. Perhaps this is because women on the pill tend to have intercourse frequently, and frequent or vigorous sex can cause cystitis.

Bones and joints

Premature closing of the epiphyses

There is a theoretical effect of oestrogen in the pill that it might stop a young girl growing. Hence the pill should normally not be given until menstrual cycles have become well and truly established, by which time a girl has almost reached her ultimate height.

The skin

Chloasma/melasma

This is a fairly common brown skin discoloration, mainly on the forehead and on each side of the face in front of the ears. It occurs during pregnancy and can also be caused by the pill. It is usually first noticed when the woman has been out in the sun. Some women also notice an increase of pigmentation in other parts of the body.

Chloasma usually fades a little when the pill is stopped but can recur with progestogen-only methods. It may never entirely disappear, because of pigment having been actually laid down in the skin. High-factor sunscreen creams can be applied, especially during the summer, and careful use of make-up when required may help.

Photosensitivity (excessive sensitivity to sunlight)

Photosensitivity is reported in pill takers, and also in women who have never been on the pill. In fact, some other medicines are a more likely cause. If it develops, skin exposed to the sun's rays develops very itchy red weals (urticaria). Treatment for this is unsatisfactory and there may be only a slight improvement if the pill is stopped. It is fairly uncommon, but it may mean that the affected woman has to avoid sunbathing altogether. Very rarely it is the first sign of one of the porphyrias.

Loss of scalp hair

Hair growth is always in balance between the growth phase and the loss phase, with different waves of each phase happening all over the head. Dermatologists consider that, in some women, the pill can do the same as happens in pregnancy. Both the pill and pregnancy can affect that balance, so that a greater proportion of the head hair than usual gets synchronized into the growth phase. This new hair inevitably comes out when the time is up for the loss phase to begin. The good news is that this problem corrects itself spontaneously, though full recovery could take a year or more.

Other side-effects

There is some weak evidence, weaker in some cases than others, for the following collection of possible side-effects: carpal tunnel syndrome, in which there is a gradual onset of tingling and pain in one or both hands; cramps and pains in the legs; gingivitis (inflammation of the gums); dry socket after tooth extraction; voice changes in singers; and Raynaud's syndrome (excessive whitening and 'deadness' of the fingers in cold weather).

7

What about blood clots, heart attacks, and strokes?

> **➲ Key points**
>
> ◆ Oestrogen in the pill increases the risk of blood clots in the arteries and veins.
> ◆ The risk is minimal for most healthy pill users.
> ◆ The risk is increased by additional risk factors, particularly smoking and high blood pressure.

A major, rare, unwanted effect of the pill is that it increases the risk of thrombosis. This means the formation of blood clots in veins and (even more rarely) arteries. But this risk should be balanced against the fact that pill users are less likely to have thrombosis than if they were pregnant. Further, this is not just a pill problem—it can also happen in women who have never taken a pill in their lives, and in men.

What causes blood clots?

Clotting is an important normal function—without the ability to clot, we would bleed to death following even a minor injury to a blood vessel. However, if blood clotting is not controlled, a clot, or thrombosis, could occur where it is *not* wanted—namely, in uninjured arteries and veins. So, to maintain good health, the body also has an effective process for getting rid of blood clots. Oestrogen in the pill increases the likelihood of clotting. Fortunately, in most healthy pill users, the clot-removing process is reset at a higher level, maintaining the balance. However, certain factors, particularly smoking, can upset this balance in favour of thrombosis.

> ## Thrombosis sounds very worrying: I am told it means clots, so does it mean that I can't use the pill if I have clots with my periods?
>
> Far from it: clots with the periods just mean that they are heavy, and could well improve dramatically if you went on the pill or the ring or patch.

Clotting in veins (venous thrombosis)

Venous thrombosis was the first clotting problem to be linked with the pill, back in 1962. It is uncommon, but when it happens it is most likely in the large veins of the leg—the so-called deep veins—where the rate of flow is slowest.

As a rule, thrombosis in a deep vein causes pain and tenderness in the calf of the affected leg, aggravated if the ankle joint is bent upwards. There may also be obvious redness and swelling on that side. Rarely, a piece of the blood clot may break off, travelling up through the heart, to finish up in the lung (*pulmonary embolism*). If the clot is big enough, this can—in around 2 per cent of cases—be fatal by stopping the blood flow through the lungs altogether. Otherwise there is breathlessness, a dry cough, and/or a sharp pain in the chest, usually on one side or the other, made worse by every breath; and sometimes a small amount of blood may be coughed up.

The treatment (apart from stopping the pill *immediately, and forever*) is usually by admission to hospital for treatment to 'thin' the blood. This is done by drugs called anti-coagulants, and by other treatments, which can dissolve or remove clots.

The effect of progestogens

Different progestogens in the pill affect the risk of a thrombosis, although the overall risk remains very tiny, whichever pill is used. The older progestogens called levonorgestrel (LNG, in Microgynon®) and norethisterone (NET, in Loestrin®), sometimes known as 'second generation' progestogens, seem to counteract some of the effects of oestrogen, including clotting. All other progestogens—the 'third generation' ones called desogestrel (DSG, in Marvelon®) and gestodene (GSD, in Femodene®) and the related ones called norgestimate (NGM, in Cilest®), drospirenone (DSP, in Yasmin® and Yaz®), and cyproterone acetate (CPA, in Dianette®)—seem not to have that effect.

All the risks are very small, and the difference between the risks of the two kinds of progestogens in the pill is especially so (Table 7.1).

To give an example, the difference between Microgynon® with LNG—the most common brand in the UK—and Marvelon® with DSG is 100 cases per million per year. Using the top estimate of 2 per cent for the risk of dying from venous thrombosis, this means the extra risk of dying from venous

Table 7.1 Risk of venous thrombosis each year per million women

Non-pill users	50–100
Women using LNG- or NET-containing pills, e.g. Microgynon 30®, Loestrin®	150
Women using other combined pills, e.g. Marvelon®, Mercilon®, Femodene®, Femodette®	250
Pregnant women	600

Source: Committee on Safety of Medicines (CSM) 2004.

thromboembolism (VTE) caused by the non-LNG non-NET pills is two per million per year. This risk difference is the same as you would get from just 2 hours of driving or 2 minutes on a motorbike.

More recent research suggests that when you look at *all* VTE cases, not just those arising in someone with another factor (see below), there may be no real difference between the types of pills. Results from the European Active Surveillance Study (EURAS) study, which observed 58 674 women for 142 475 woman-years, showed that although pill users had a higher risk of venous thrombosis compared with non-pill users, the rate was the same for all the combined oral contraceptives studied.

Whatever the added risk from the pill may be, it is not worse with increasing duration of use, and goes away within 4 weeks of stopping the pill.

Other risk factors for venous thrombosis

It's not just the pill that affects the risk of venous thrombosis. The most important background factors that make clotting in veins more likely are shown in Box 7.1.

Box 7.1 Risk factors for venous thrombosis

- Dehydration.
- Immobile or very sedentary.
- Long-haul journeys, often but not only by aeroplane.
- Obesity, high BMI (see Glossary).
- Smoking.
- Surgery (especially affecting the leg)—or a leg fracture.
- Pregnancy and delivery.
- Family history.
- Blood group A, B, or AB.

Being overweight or smoking are particularly important modifiable risks. In the EURAS study, obese women (BMI more than 30) had an approximately threefold higher thrombosis risk compared with women with normal weight (BMI 20.0–24.9).

I am going on a long scheduled flight to Australia. I am on the pill: are there any precautions I should take?

High altitude and sitting down for a long time increase the risk of thrombosis, although this has only been shown in women with pre-existing conditions that themselves increase the risk. However, since few women flying will know ahead of time that they have these conditions, it is sensible to take simple precautions. Take a maximum amount of fluid and a minimum of caffeine and alcohol, which cause the kidney to produce more urine: the risk is greater if you are dehydrated. If you are at all overweight, even though not exactly glamorous, it is a good idea to use special below-knee support stockings.

There is usually no need actually to come off the pill—many flight attendants use it all the time. But follow their example and take some exercise during the flight by walking around the plane every hour or so.

Clotting in arteries (arterial thrombosis)

The main reason why arterial thrombosis occurs is atherosclerosis ('hardening of the arteries'). It affects almost everyone in due course, including women who have never taken a single pill in their lives and *men*, usually at a younger age than women.

In the more developed countries of the world it has usually started even before the age of 20, and gets more marked as the individual gets older, especially if he or she is a smoker. It affects some much more than others, and one important factor seems to be high levels or an abnormal ratio of the levels of the various blood fats.

Changes in blood-clotting factors, especially those which affect the blood platelets, are also important. Once the walls of an artery have been damaged by atherosclerosis, clotting on the surface of the roughened bit of the wall can then occur and eventually this may block up the artery altogether. If this occurs in an artery supplying the heart muscle, it causes a heart attack (coronary thrombosis). If in the brain, it can lead to a stroke (cerebral thrombosis).

What factors affect arterial thrombosis risk?

The risk of arterial thrombosis is very low in women of childbearing age. Although the pill can increase the risk of cerebral thrombosis, the actual number of women who have a stroke on the pill is extremely small. The good news is that all the recent studies have found that the pill does not increase the risk of coronary thrombosis at all, unless the woman is a smoker, or has one of the other recognized 'risk factors' discussed in Box 7.2.

Box 7.2 Risk factors for arterial thrombosis

- Cigarette smoking, especially if heavy. Coronary thrombosis in otherwise healthy women before the menopause is almost exclusively an illness of smokers.
- Diabetes, whether type 1 or type 2 controlled by diet or tablets.
- Family history.
- High blood pressure.
- High cholesterol (LDL not HDL) or triglycerides.
- Increasing age, especially beyond 35 in smokers.
- Migraine with aura.
- Obesity, high BMI (see Glossary).
- Blood group A, B, or AB.

Blood pressure and the pill

In most pill users there is a measurable slight rise in blood pressure. However, in only about one woman out of every 100 who takes modern pills does this reach the level at which doctors term it hypertension. The reason why the rest are not more affected is still not clear. Some individuals are known to be more prone generally to raised blood pressure: those with a family history, those who have had kidney disease, and some black people. The pill may 'bring out' the blood pressure problem in such women, particularly as they get older. One group of researchers has also shown that women with hypertension on the pill have higher levels of the hormone ethinylestradiol (EE) in their blood than other pill-users. So perhaps the few individuals who develop this problem are exceptional in the way their bodies absorb and handle the pill's hormones.

Whatever the reason, there are two main points about raised blood pressure. First, it usually does *not* make you feel at all unwell. Secondly, when large groups of both men and women with even very mild hypertension have been followed up, they have not remained as healthy over the years as comparison groups with entirely normal blood pressure readings. Blood pressure seems to be linked with nearly all the diseases of the circulatory system and is often a feature of people who later suffer thrombosis in veins, heart attacks, and strokes. It also has the risk itself of becoming uncontrollable, even with drugs, leading to malignant hypertension, which is very rare but fatal.

If the pill was the cause, just stopping the pill generally brings the blood pressure back to normal within a month or two. All brands of the combined pill tend to cause a recurrence of the problem, and so should be avoided, but progestogen-only methods may be tried, often successfully.

Minimizing risk

If you have high cholesterol in your family, or you are unlucky enough to have diabetes, or have now developed high blood pressure, you can benefit from taking dietary advice and treatment, managing your stress levels, and increasing physical exercise. If you are overweight you ought to be able to return to the ideal weight for your height (BMI less than 30 or, better, less than 25) by diet plus exercise—and this is well worth doing anyway. But the number one risk factor that you can do something about is *smoking*.

Smoking in effect ages your arteries. The pill's hazards are heavily concentrated in cigarette smokers, particularly as they get older. Not only does smoking increase the risk of arterial disease, it also makes the attack more likely to be fatal. On top of that, smokers are at greater risk of bronchitis, cancer of the lung, larynx, bladder, and cervix, reduced fertility, and even gangrene of the legs. If you add the pill to your cigarettes, you make smoking even more dangerous than it would otherwise be. In contrast, if you don't smoke there is no demonstrable effect of the pill at all on arterial disease risk.

These facts, plus a greater understanding of the benefits of the pill for older women, mean that for women free of all risk factors, including excess weight and smoking, there need no longer be any upper age limit for the pill. *But* the upper age limit for heavy smokers is 35 years.

The obvious action is to stop smoking—*research shows it is always worth giving up*. After a few years ex-smokers have no greater chance of dying than lifetime non-smokers. By stopping smoking they even benefit those around them.

8

What about cancer?

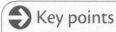 **Key points**

◆ Overall, pill users are less likely to get cancer than non-users.

◆ You are less likely to get cancer of the ovaries, or cancer of the uterus, bowel, or rectum if you take the pill.

◆ There is no increase in lung cancer or melanoma.

◆ The pill does not appear to increase the overall risk of breast cancer, although some uncertainty remains.

◆ Long-term use of the pill (more than 8 years) slightly increases the risk of cervical cancer, though it is almost eliminated by having regular smears.

Ever since the pill was first marketed there has always been a concern that it might be found to increase the risk of some types of cancer. But cancers may not develop until after many years—up to 30 years—of exposure to any cancer-producing agent. Since the pill has now been around for over 40 years, we are beginning to obtain useful information about possible links between it and some forms of cancer.

In view of the widespread nature of the pill's effects, we should not be too surprised if it can in fact modify the risk either way: promoting some cancers but actually reducing the likelihood of other types. As in the scales of Figure 8.1, research suggests that the good effects tend to slightly outweigh the bad. If the pill increases the risk of any cancer, the harmful effect is likely (not certain) to be greater the longer the pill is used, and might persist for a few years in ex-users. In contrast, if the pill reduces a risk, as it does for cancer of the ovary and endometrium, the protective effect is definitely greater the longer the duration of use, and continues among ex-users.

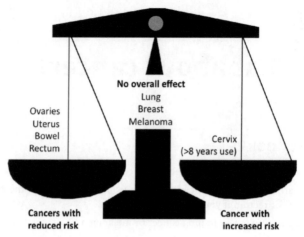

Figure 8.1 Cancer and the pill: a balance.

The breast

Breast cancer is the most common cancer in UK women. During the four decades that the pill has been available, breast cancer rates have risen and one in nine women will develop breast cancer at some point in their lives. It is tempting to conclude that the pill is to blame. However, statistics show a rise in breast cancer in all age groups, and the greatest rise among older women who never had a chance to take the pill. With such a high rate of this disease it must inevitably be expected to happen in women whether they took the pill or not. Regardless of the pill, there have also been increasing rates of several well-known breast cancer risk factors (Box 8.1).

> ## Box 8.1 Known risk factors for breast cancer
>
> ◆ Young age at the first menstrual period.
>
> ◆ Late age at the menopause.
>
> ◆ Delayed first child to after age 30.
>
> ◆ Family history of a close relative (mother or sister) with breast cancer, especially if it was diagnosed under age 40.
>
> ◆ Obesity.
>
> ◆ Possibly, high-fat diets.
>
> ◆ Possibly, drugs such as antibiotics; or other modern-day pollutants of air, water, or food.
>
> ◆ Increasing age—the strongest risk factor (in England the risk of developing breast cancer is one in 1900 up to age 30; one in 50 up to age 50).

In 1996, the Collaborative Group on Hormonal Factors in Breast Cancer reanalysed data from over 53 000 women with breast cancer and over 100 000 controls without it, from 54 studies in 25 countries. This research suggested a very small risk as a result of taking the pill in current users, but this risk completely disappeared in ex-users. The latest research has been more reassuring, with two large studies showing no difference in risk between ever users of the pill (current and past) and never users in their risk of breast cancer.

What does all this mean for women taking the pill?

If present at all, risk is minimal and should not pose a great concern to healthy pill users. In addition, cancer diagnosed among pill takers tends to be less advanced than in women not taking the pill. Certainly there is no evidence to suggest that risk is increased by:

- Past use of the pill.
- Starting the pill as a teenager.
- Using it before the first pregnancy.
- Duration of use.
- Dose or type of hormone in the particular pill.

Until we are completely sure about the risks, some people may prefer to switch to a different method at about the age (35 or so) when the background cancer risk begins to rise. Methods such as the IUD (no hormones) or IUS (minimal hormones) are worth considering.

The cervix

Cancer of the cervix is really an STI. It is associated with a virus or a combination of viruses (particularly the HPV types16 and18) that are transmitted sexually. The risk for an unprotected woman with many sexual partners can be many times that of a one-man woman whose partner is a one-woman man. Barrier methods such as condoms are protective, and cervical cancer vaccines are also now available, which protect against the high-risk strains of HPV.

Research suggests that the pill is not the cause of this cancer but may act as a co-factor. Cigarette smoking acts even more strongly as a co-factor. Co-factors seem to *promote the abnormal cell changes once they have been started* and so speed the transition through all the stages of pre-cancer of what is called cervical intraepithelial neoplasia (CIN). CIN can be picked up from cervical smears and then eradicated, if found. So pill users (like all women) should be sure to have regular cervical smears, 3-yearly from the age of 25 onwards, with extra tests as advised if any abnormal cells have been found. Even in smokers and pill takers, 3-yearly is sufficiently often for early changes to be treated and prevent cervical cancer.

The uterus: the endometrium

Good news! Several studies show that risk of cancer of the endometrium (the lining of the womb) is halved if the pill is taken for at least 1 year, with a three-fold reduction after 5 years. This *protective effect* has now been confirmed by many other studies, and encouragingly seems to persist in ex-users—for 15 years, possibly even longer.

The ovary

Even better news! More than 10 large studies consistently report a clear-cut protective effect, which is again greater the longer the pill has been used. This is really important, since this cancer kills more than any other gynaecological malignancy. After 5 years there is a threefold reduction in the risk, and protection continues among ex-users for at least 15–30 years, maybe even for life.

Choriocarcinoma and trophoblastic disease

Sometimes there is complete failure of the normal development of a pregnancy, resulting in trophoblastic disease. This produces large amounts of the special pregnancy hormone hCG. This is not itself a cancer, but has a very small risk of turning into one. The pill does not make the original trophoblastic disease more likely to happen, but if the pill is taken before the hCG level in the blood has declined to zero, some research suggests that cancer risk may be doubled. Hence, in the UK, hormonal contraception is usually avoided until the hCG test is back to normal.

Colon and rectum (bowel cancer)

Several studies have now confirmed that pill takers are less likely to develop cancers of the large bowel and rectum, although the reasons for this are not fully understood. Good news again since, after breast cancer, bowel cancers as a group are the next most common cancers in women.

9

Who can take the pill, who can't, and who needs careful monitoring?

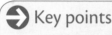 Key points

◆ Most women *can* take the pill.

◆ Conditions that increase the risk of blood clots, affect the liver, or which may be worsened by additional hormones may mean that a different method of contraception should be considered.

◆ If you have just one minor risk factor, it may still be possible to take the pill.

◆ Combinations of risk factors mean that risks of using the pill outweigh the benefits and an alternative method of contraception should be used.

As you've seen in previous chapters, the pill is safe for the majority of women, but for others the balance of risks outweighs the benefits. If you answer 'yes' to any of the questions in Box 9.1, you will know from Chapters 7 and 8 that the risks of taking the pill outweigh the potential benefits and you should use a different method of contraception, at least until the risk factor goes away (e.g. more than 3 weeks since having a baby or losing weight to a BMI of 29 or less).

But what about women who don't respond 'yes' to the questions in Box 9.1, but who are not completely fit and healthy. Can they take the pill? The answer is very individual and depends on the extent to which their personal or family history and their lifestyle affects the risks of using the pill, or if they have any medical conditions or take any medication that might be affected by the hormones in the pill. An important point to understand is that if you have more than one risk factor, there is a dramatic increase in risk (Box 9.2).

Box 9.1 Screening checklist for the COC

- Do you think you might already be pregnant?
- Have you had a baby in the last 3 weeks?
- Do you have heart disease?
- Have you ever had a heart attack or a stroke?
- Do you take medicine for high cholesterol?
- Have you ever had a blood clot in a leg (venous thrombosis) or your lungs (pulmonary embolism)?
- Do you have high blood pressure (more than 160/95—either number)?
- Do you smoke *and* are over 35?
- Do you have diabetes affecting the eyes, kidneys, arteries, or nerves?
- Do you have, or have you ever had, migraine *with* aura (typically visual symptoms which last up to an hour and resolve *before or as* a migraine headache starts)?
- Do you have active liver disease?
- Are you overweight (BMI above 30 (see Glossary)) *and* aged over 35 or have a BMI of 40 or above at any age?
- Do you have breast cancer?
- Do you have ongoing gall bladder disease?

Box 9.2 How risk factors multiply

Consider a healthy 25-year-old woman who is not a diabetic, has normal blood fat levels and blood pressure, and does not smoke. If she starts to smoke cigarettes her chances of a coronary are around three times greater than before, depending on how many she smokes. If she swallows a daily pill and also smokes more than 15 cigarettes a day, her risk goes up by at most two for the pill *multiplied* by three (for the smoking), to six times the initial value. Double that if her daily consumption is 30 cigarettes. What would happen if she had a third risk factor, say a sufficiently raised blood pressure to add a further five-times risk? Multiplying again, she would then be five times 12 or up to 60 times less safe than a healthy non-smoker with normal blood pressure not taking the pill.

Note: all these figures are very approximate.

The bottom line is, **if you have more than one risk factor, you should not use the pill.** But you can still have effective contraception—see Chapters 3 and 17.

If you have only one risk factor, that in itself does not contraindicate the pill; you usually need to be monitored carefully and should be ready to discontinue the pill should the condition worsen, or a new risk factor or relevant disease appear.

Conditions that increase the risk of blood clots

Heart disease

The question to ask the doctor is: 'Is there is an added risk of thrombosis?' *Structural heart disease* (meaning significant heart valve trouble or so-called shunts and septal defects), in which the heart's anatomy has not been completely restored to normal by surgery, usually means that the pill should not be used. Also important here are diseases called *pulmonary hypertension*; an irregular heartbeat problem where clots can be formed called *atrial fibrillation*; and any *cyanotic heart disease* (meaning the patient's lips are blue all the time). Mild disorders, such as *mitral valve prolapse* or successfully repaired *atrial septal defects*, do not affect use of the pill.

Past history of any form of thrombosis

The pill should be avoided whenever clotting in any artery or vein anywhere in the body has occurred. It makes no difference whether it occurred in a situation that makes clotting more likely, such as pregnancy or being confined to bed after an operation, or was completely unexpected. All of these troubles are rare, but the least uncommon would be clotting in one of the leg veins.

A family history of venous thrombosis

You may not be able to take the pill if a thrombosis or VTE occurred in a parent, brother, or sister under the age of 45, particularly if it happened in them 'out of the blue' rather than because of a recognized cause such as being immobilized. If available, blood tests for *hereditary* trouble such as Factor V Leiden should be done. If any tests are positive for increased risk—or if the tests are not (yet) available—you should not take the pill.

If your results are completely normal, you definitely can take the pill. However, you are not completely risk free, since there are some hereditary changes in the blood which modern testing still cannot detect.

Can I take a combined pill, patch, or ring if I have varicose veins?

On their own these rarely mean that you must avoid the method, provided that you have not suffered from clotting within them. If you have them badly and have suffered a condition called phlebitis in them in the past, it is better to use a different method. The pill should not be taken while you are actually having either medical or surgical treatment for varicose veins—see below.

A family history of arterial disease: a heart attack (coronary thrombosis) or stroke

This means again that the history was in a parent, brother, or sister under the age of 45 who was not a heavy smoker, a diabetic, overweight, or suffering from high blood pressure. In the absence of these well-known risk factors to explain their problem, tests for fasting blood lipids (fats) should be arranged to check if you have an inherited cause. If they show levels which the lab says make you especially prone to heart disease or a stroke, then you should avoid the combined pill altogether or it *might* be allowed with careful monitoring.

If your own levels of the various lipids they test are normal then, despite the family history, you can be pretty confident there is no hereditary problem and the pill is OK to use.

I have angina: does this mean I can't take the pill?

Angina means heart pain, of a type, which is usually described as a heavy feeling behind the chest bone or tightness around the chest, and perhaps going up the neck or down the arms, which is brought on by exercise. If this diagnosis has been given to such a pain, it means that the heart muscle is being temporarily supplied with too little blood. This happens because the coronary (heart) arteries are already affected by atherosclerosis, i.e. hardening of the arteries. So to reduce the chances of an actual coronary thrombosis, which would block the arteries altogether, the pill is certainly best avoided by any woman who has been told she has angina.

Diabetes

Diseases of the circulation are already more likely in diabetics. Women who have diabetes severely, with signs of damage to the arteries, nerves, or kidneys, or changes affecting the eye should definitely not take the pill. However, some young diabetics who are free of any signs of complications of the disease may take the combined pill for a limited time because they need maximum protection against pregnancy. If the POP or non-hormonal methods are not satisfactory alternatives, the lowest effective dose of pill is an option, with careful monitoring. It is especially crazy for diabetics to smoke—if they do they certainly should not use the pill.

Women with a strong family history of diabetes, or who are overweight, or who had the very mild blood test changes of diabetes in pregnancy, or who gave birth to a baby weighing more than 4.5 kg all need to be carefully observed on the pill. Sometimes a special 'glucose tolerance test' may be arranged. But the main thing by far, if any of those factors apply to you—or if you have PCOS, which has connections with diabetes—is to lose weight and certainly not put more on!

High blood pressure

Repeated readings at or above 160/95 are too high both for starting and for continuing with the pill. If there is a past history of blood pressure going up very significantly on the pill, and returning to normal when it was stopped, this also means that the pill should be avoided in future. Everything depends on the actual levels. Readings up to and around 140/90 normally just indicate the need for frequent check-ups. If you have higher levels your doctor may advise you to switch to a progestogen-only or non-hormonal method. It is important to remember that a rise in blood pressure can be an early warning sign of a circulatory disease. So if there are other risk factors already, such as smoking, even a small rise can be important. *It is obviously vital, therefore, if you use the pill, that you have your blood pressure taken regularly.*

Cigarette smoking and age

Smokers should generally stop the pill at 35. Although some authorities allow light smokers to continue to use the pill into their 40s, another method definitely would be preferred. Non-smokers, if 100 per cent free of all the risk factors listed here, may continue to take the pill, right up to age 51. It would be even safer, overall, to switch to a long-acting method like an IUD or IUS.

I smoke at least 20 cigarettes a day: how can I stop?

In Britain, ASH (Action on Smoking and Health—http://www.ash.co.uk) can give you loads of practical advice and there may be an anti-smoking clinic you could attend locally. Quitline is particularly useful (0800 002200). Smoking substitutes give your body the powerful (as strong as heroin) drug of addiction it so craves, in a much cleaner way than along with all that carbon monoxide and carcinogenic tar. Some find the nicotine inhaler good, as it gives you something to do with your hands.

But there is no magic method and you will never succeed unless:

- You really want to give up.
- You are prepared to work hard to do so.
- You get your partner to join you if they are a smoker.

Excessive weight

The BMI is calculated as a person's weight in kilograms divided by his or her height in metres, squared. For good general health, your BMI should be between 19 and 25. Excessive weight increases the risk of both venous and arterial thrombosis, so a woman with a BMI of 40 or above should not take the pill. If the BMI is between 26 and 30 the pill can be used. If the BMI is over 30, the pill should only be used if no alternative methods suit. Since the venous thrombosis risk takes priority with high BMI, a non-oestrogen-dominant pill (containing LNG or NET—see Chapter 16) should normally be used.

> ## Does it affect my choice of pill that I am very underweight?
>
> Underweight women (with a BMI below 19) are more likely to have side-effects such as menstrual cramps, nausea, and breast discomfort, and to have a long delay in return of their periods after stopping the pill. Hence they should try either a combined pill with the lowest possible dose, or perhaps the POP.

Migraine

Migraine *without* aura (typically episodic 'sick' headaches) does not appear to increase the risk of thrombosis and the pill is safe to use. Attacks often occur in the pill-free week as the drop in oestrogen can be a trigger.

> ## Box 9.3 Migraine in the 'pill-free' week
>
> If migraine without aura occurs predictably in the pill-free week, there are several solutions:
>
> 1. Take any ultra-low-dose monophasic combined pill on the tricycle basis described in Chapter 12 or even take the pill continuously 365/365 (Chapter 12). For this purpose, choose a pill from as near as possible to the bottom of one of the 'ladders' (Chapter 16, Fig. 16.1).
>
> 2. Change to a progestogen-only method that also stops ovulation, such as Cerazette® or Depo-Provera®.
>
> 3. Continue your combined pill in the usual way, but ask your doctor about using 100 mcg oestrogen *patches* to apply to your skin during the pill-free week.

In contrast, migraine *with* aura is associated with increased risk of stroke. Although there is no evidence that aura itself causes stroke, this type of migraine acts as a 'marker' that the person has a higher risk of stroke. So it makes sense to avoid anything that has an additional risk. For this reason, migraine *with* aura means that you should never go on the pill, and you should stop the pill if you develop these attacks. It is possible to have a trial of the pill if you had migraine *with* aura more than 5 years earlier or only during pregnancy, but it should be stopped immediately if aura develops.

The word 'aura' is used for strange symptoms, nearly always (99 per cent of cases) affecting the eyes: typically visual disturbances in part of the field of vision on the same side in both eyes. People tend to think at first that it's in one of their eyes, but if they cover up each in turn they discover that the aura affects part of what each eye sees. Funny sensations may also happen, in about one-third of cases, but nearly always there is something affecting the eyes as well. There could be pins and needles spreading up one arm or one side of the face or the tongue. Some notice a particular disturbance of speech: they find it temporarily impossible to say the names of things, objects that they know perfectly well.

Much more serious, though not aura, is sudden blindness in one eye, or loss of muscle power or sensation affecting the leg as well as the arm on one side. These suggest a thrombosis has actually happened and would be reasons for stopping the pill immediately and going straight to the emergency department of a hospital.

How can I be sure if it's aura?

Symptoms last up to an hour, typically around 20–30 minutes, and resolve just *before* or shortly after the headache starts. Often there is a bright zig-zag line which gradually enlarges to form a bright C-shape surrounding the blank area of lost vision. If asked to draw what they see, people with true aura inevitably wave their hand beside their head and/or draw a zig-zag line in the air on the same side as their visual disturbance. The ensuing headache may be as bad as in migraine without aura, but can be very mild or even absent. Aura symptoms should also not be confused with *premonitory symptoms* that some people get a day or so beforehand: these can take the form of unusual tiredness or cravings for certain foods (including chocolate!). Light sensitivity (light bothering you more than usual) or generalized eye blurring or other eye symptoms occurring before and containing into the headache–or only happening during the headache–are not typical of mygraine aura.

Other conditions increasing the risk of thrombosis

These include

- Surgical removal of the spleen if the number of platelets is way above normal (>500 × 10^9/L).
- Connective tissue diseases, such as SLE and polyarteritis nodosa.
- Some blood diseases—leukaemia, polycythaemia.

Life circumstances that increase the risk of thrombosis

Immobilization in bed, such as after an accident

This means stopping the pill at once, since being immobile in bed, perhaps in a plaster cast, increases the risk of leg thrombosis. Even having just one limb immobilized, say after a fracture, might lead to thrombosis locally in that limb, so the pill may need stopping even if you are not confined to bed. Disabled women who are *confined to a wheelchair* may be permitted to take a non-oestrogen-dominant (LNG or NET), preferably 20 mcg, combined pill provided they are not also overweight, and with special care and counselling.

Surgery

I am going into hospital for an operation—should I stop the pill?

You should stop the pill if it is *any* treatment for varicose veins, or *any* operation on the legs (including arthroscopy), or you are told the operation somewhere else in the body will last for more than 30 minutes and you will be confined to bed for at least the first 24 hours.

If you need to stop the pill, you should stop it at least 4 weeks before surgery and use a different method of contraception. Progestogen-only methods are not thought to affect clotting factors to any important extent, and can be continued up to and after major or leg operations. One of these methods (e.g. Cerazette®) could be ideal to tide you over the whole time on the waiting list, in hospital, and until you restart the combined pill.

You can restart the pill at least 2 weeks following full mobility after the operation. If you have not had sex, you can use the 'quick start' method (Chapter 12) with precautions for seven more days. Otherwise start on day 1 of the next period.

If you go into hospital for a planned major operation without having stopped the pill, you may be given heparin, a blood-thinning drug. Heparin is also given if you have emergency surgery, so always inform the surgeon if you are on the pill.

Does being sterilized count as a major operation?

Not if done by modern laparoscopy techniques. Therefore, there is no need to stop any of the combined hormonal methods, and usually it is best to continue after the operation until the end of the current packet/cycle of treatment. The POP is continued for at least 7 days and usually until the next period.

Travel to high altitudes

All women travelling to above 2500 m and especially above 4000 m should be informed about the risk of altitude sickness. This happens in some people unpredictably and is not caused by the pill, but in its most severe forms thrombosis can happen. As a general rule the pill is perhaps best not used. Yet it is not ruled out, and a healthy woman trekking the Himalayas could use the pill if she planned always to follow the golden rule: 'climb high but sleep low'.

Conditions affected by the pill hormones

Gallstones

If these have been treated medically in the past they could recur, so it would normally be best to avoid the pill in future unless there is no suitable alternative. The pill can be used if the gall bladder has been completely removed.

Liver disease

If you have any illness that affects liver function causing jaundice, then the pill, like alcohol, should be avoided. This is normally for 3 months after the relevant blood tests have become normal. Further tests of liver function may be advised after a month or so of pill taking.

Breast cancer

Women being treated for breast cancer should not take the pill. Occasionally, the pill is used by women who have been successfully treated for breast cancer in the past, but only if there is no suitable alternative.

If a woman has a mutated form of one of the genes known to be involved in breast cancer (*BRCA1* or *2*), the pill can be used, with caution. It's worth noting the women with these mutated genes are also at higher risk of ovarian cancer. Since the pill very effectively reduces this risk, there may be an argument for taking the pill.

If you had a minor operation in the past for a lump or lumpiness in the breast, ask whether it is advisable to continue with or start taking the pill. If the laboratory found any tissue with what is called epithelial atypia (abnormal cells), in that unusual case the pill really would be best avoided altogether. Otherwise this *personal* history is of minimal concern.

Family history?

If breast cancer affected a relative under age 40, the pill *may* be used, probably starting with the lowest dose of oestrogen available (20 mcg), with extra counselling about the pros and cons and then reassessment every 5 years or so. If the cancer occurred in an older close relative, there is no restriction on use of the pill.

Inflammatory bowel diseases (Crohn's disease and ulcerative colitis)

These uncommon but unpleasant bowel diseases cause pain and diarrhoea. In some research the diseases were more common in pill-takers. But in a large group of patients whose disease was well controlled with treatment, the women on the pill were no more likely to suffer flare-ups than the others. So that means the benefits outweigh any risks of taking the pill, generally.

A complication affecting the liver called *sclerosing cholangitis* or *hepatitis* means the pill should not be used. Also, if any patient gets a bad attack of bowel trouble itself, needing hospitalization, there is an increased risk of thrombosis. So the pill should be stopped and for as long as the disease is severe. If all went well thereafter she could use it again, with caution.

Despite the diarrhoea, the hormones are usually absorbed normally, so there is no need to take a stronger brand. Absorption could be affected in one of the conditions (Crohn's disease) if it badly affects the small bowel—meaning a non-oral method (injection, implant, IUD, or IUS) would be preferable.

Past history of any serious condition occurring or worsening in a previous pregnancy and/or known to be affected by pill hormones

Chorea is a rare condition that causes the patient to make strange uncontrolled fidgety movements of the head, arms, and legs. It may have occurred in the past, during an attack of rheumatic fever or in pregnancy. With or without such a history, it has been found to happen in one or two pill users. It generally seems to clear up if the pill is discontinued (and usually avoided in future).

Other skin conditions such as *pemphigoid gestationis* and the severe skin rash *erythema multiforme* are also adversely affected by the pill.

Idiopathic intracranial hypertension, previously known as 'pseudo-tumour cerebri' or 'benign intracranial hypertension', is a rare condition of headache and loss of vision, which can imitate a brain tumour. It is not as benign for the eyesight as its previous name suggests. It typically affects young women who are very overweight. Other drugs can cause it, and cases occurring in pill takers are not necessarily caused by the pill. However, it certainly might be to blame when, after investigation, the real problem is found to be thrombosis of certain important veins in the brain. In either type, urgent treatment is needed. Specialists recommend that all types of contraceptive hormone treatment should be avoided (even the progestogen-only methods).

Other medical conditions

Age above 51

Not exactly an illness but safer options are available which by that age (the average age of the menopause) are equally effective. So it is hardly sensible to take the risks of the pill since they go up steadily with age.

Recent abnormal vaginal bleeding, other than at period times, from the uterus until its cause has been found

The reason for avoiding the pill here is that any vaginal bleeding that is not clearly connected with periods—especially if it happens after intercourse—must be diagnosed as quickly as possible. This is to rule out disease of the uterus and cervix, commonly non-malignant growths called polyps, but very, very rarely cancer. As irregular bleeding of the type known as BTB can occur on the pill, if this rule were not followed there is a risk that the diagnosis would be delayed, because the bleeding might be thought to be a side-effect of the pill. However, once the gynaecologist has definitely ruled out a serious cause for the abnormal bleeding, they will almost certainly then be happy for you to take the pill.

Actual or possible pregnancy

Here the main reason for avoiding the pill until pregnancy has been ruled out is that there is a possible risk, though if it exists it must be very, very small, that pill taking during pregnancy might damage the baby.

Scanty or very irregular periods or their absence (amenorrhoea)

There used to be anxiety about this and taking the pill. But now—after any investigation that may be needed has been done—do not be surprised if the pill is recommended. You may be short of oestrogen and the pill is an excellent source of that along with contraception. If you have no need for contraception, oestrogen from HRT may be offered.

In teenagers, starting the pill should always be delayed until periods have started. Otherwise there are no proven special medical risks at this age.

Prolactinoma

This disorder of the pituitary gland is a cause of infertility and so a rare reason for even thinking about going on the pill. The woman concerned should already be seeing a specialist, and once treatment begins pregnancy is very possible. UK experts allow use of the pill but only while taking the treatment and supervised by a specialist.

Previous failure of the pill (pregnancy while taking it)

The answer, especially if you keep missing tablets, is most often to try an 'unforgettable' method such as the injection or implant, or an IUD or the IUS.

But your very ability to get pregnant by missing an occasional pill (lots of people do forget and get away with it) may mean you are someone whose metabolism gets rid of the pill hormones from your body extra rapidly. To improve your 'margin for error' you could tricycle the pill or take it continuously 365/365 (see Chapter 12). This means fewer of those pill-free breaks, which are times of potential weakness as a contraceptive.

Abnormal cervical smears under observation or treated

The pill may definitely continue to be used as the woman's choice during investigation for an abnormality in a cervical smear test, or following successful treatment whether by the laser or large-loop excision or a cone biopsy (removal of the affected skin under anaesthetic). All experts agree that attending without fail for follow-up smears as instructed is the first priority. This gives such safe monitoring of the situation that, if a woman wants to continue taking the pill, she may certainly do so. She might decide after full discussion to use a male or female barrier method in future (as well, or instead): this would have the advantage of protecting the cervix from the virus causing the abnormal cells. The choice is up to her—it would be even more important to stop smoking!

Melanoma

Melanoma is a cancer that can develop from a mole, one of those black patches which people have on their skin. The change to cancer is more likely in skin exposed to a lot of sunlight. Most experts think the pill does *not* promote this cancer. Hence anyone who is given this diagnosis while taking the pill may stay on it if she so wishes, or even start using the method for the first time.

Chronic (long-term) diseases

Epilepsy

The pill does not cause epilepsy. In fact many sufferers report fewer attacks when they go on the pill, especially if their attacks tend to come on either pre- or during periods in their normal cycles. However, a very few do get more frequent epileptic attacks, and may have to give up the method. There is also the distinct possibility that the tablets they take to control fits may interfere with the hormones of the pill once absorbed into the body, and reduce the protection it provides against pregnancy (see Chapter 15 for what to do).

Asthma

Some women, especially those whose asthma is always worse premenstrually, notice that their symptoms are improved on the pill. In a few, they are worsened, maybe because of the pill affecting an allergic factor in the asthma. In the majority there is no change. So the pill is an appropriate choice in asthma.

Thyroid disease

Research suggests that the pill may actually protect against thyroid disease. This beneficial effect of the pill seems to apply to both overactivity and underactivity of the gland.

Sickle cell anaemia

This type of anaemia affects only black people. Of the two forms, the milder, more common one, called *sickle cell trait*, poses no problem for pill taking. In the past, patients with the rarer *sickle cell anaemia* were told the pill must be avoided. During the painful attacks (so-called crises), damaged red blood cells block up tiny arteries in the body. Theoretically these attacks might be worsened by oestrogen in the pill, promoting thrombosis and thus turning temporary blockages of the microcirculation into more permanent ones. However, other evidence suggests that the progestogen of the pill might have good effects. Since pregnancy is particularly dangerous in this condition, many experts allow a low-dose, non-oestrogen-dominant pill to be used, after full discussion. But it is more usual to prescribe Depo-Provera®, which has the benefit of reducing the frequency of painful crises.

Are there any special considerations for people with a long-term illness?

Discuss this with your doctor, who should consider particularly whether there is an additive or multiplying effect between effects of the disease and of the pill. Thus if the disease makes thrombosis more likely anyway, special blood tests may be necessary. It may be better to use a method other than the pill or, in lesser cases, the pill can be taken with careful monitoring. In the latter, it is a matter of balancing known and potential unknown risks of the pill in your total situation against those of pregnancy and the pros and cons of alternative methods. Be sure that a doctor or specialist who knows the full story follows you up.

Part 3

Taking the pill

10

How do I get the pill?

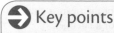

Key points

- The pill is available from general practitioners' surgeries and specialized community centres.
- The appointment is completely confidential, even if you are under age.

Before deciding whether the pill is right for you, you need to know where to turn for advice. Everyone should have access to someone, usually a doctor or a nurse trained in family planning, who can answer your questions about contraception and go over every aspect that applies to you personally. The main choice is between a local community clinic and general practice.

Details of community family-planning clinics in the UK can be found on http://www.yell.com and through the Family Planning Association (FPA) (http://www.fpa.org.uk or call 0845 122 8690). If you choose to go to one of them, you do not need to bring a doctor's letter with you. Most clinics have no objection if you take a partner, friend, or relative with you. They are usually staffed by healthcare professionals who work solely in women's healthcare and who can offer more than just help to avoid unwanted pregnancy. For a start, they are also very ready to help those who are a bit late with a period and think they might already be pregnant. If a urine test shows that you are in fact pregnant, clinics can arrange appropriate counselling about the pregnancy. Most family-planning nurses and doctors are easy to talk to, and are very helpful if you have emotional problems or difficulties with any aspect of sex. Special counselling can be arranged for couples where sex has become a problem. At major centres there are also readily available services for screening, health education, testing for STIs, male and female sterilization—in short a 'seamless' well-woman/well-man service.

Your family doctor can also provide contraception. The visits may be briefer than community clinics, partly because he or she probably knows most of the important medical facts about you already. It is entirely up to you whether you prefer to go to a clinic or to your doctor's—or any neighbouring doctor's—surgery. Some practices now run at least one special or 'dedicated' family-planning session each week.

> ## What shall I do if I need some more pills (or any hormonal method) when in a foreign country?
>
> Look up your variety of pill or the other method on the website http://www. ippf.org.uk. You should then be able to use the name of the nearest equivalent, locally available brand when you visit the doctor or a chemist.

What happens at the first visit?

The receptionist will take your name, date of birth, and contact details. A nurse or doctor will take more confidential details in the consulting room. There is usually a standard card with specific questions to answer. *As a minimum* you should always be asked some questions about your medical history and aspects of your family history in order to establish that you are suitable for the pill. Your age and smoking habits should be noted as well as your general health, and then if you have had an abortion or miscarriage or ever had treatment for an STI. You should be weighed and have your blood pressure checked.

To help you make your decision about which method of contraception suits you, the staff will describe and discuss the various methods, and answer any questions that you have. If there are any special points—for instance, if you are a smoker over 35, or are uneasy and unsure about things, or are under age 16— then time should be made for a longer discussion on all the pros and cons.

Will I be examined?

An examination is *not* a vital part of the first visit to start on the pill—apart from checking blood pressure (which is indeed something you should insist on having done). Otherwise, you only need to be examined if you have noticed any changes or abnormalities, such as breast lumps or a vaginal discharge.

Cervical smear tests are recommended in all sexually active women aged 25–65. They are now recommended 3-yearly till aged 50 and 5-yearly up to 65, but stopping then (or by 60 in Scotland). However, especially if you have not yet started having intercourse, or are anxious about examination, there is absolutely no need for it just because of the pill.

They have asked me to come back for a smear test in only 6 months. What does this mean? Can I continue on the pill?

No reason to panic. It may be because the first test picked up too few of the right kind of cells for the lab to check they were completely normal, so they want to look again. Or, some abnormal cells were found on the smear. Quite often these are got rid of by the body without any further treatment anyway, and so are not seen when you have the repeat done. If the repeat smear shows persistent abnormalities, the doctor or nurse will discuss the whole matter with you. He or she will explain that even persistent changes in the smear can be readily dealt with, and actual cancer of the cervix—which in any case would not occur for many years—can be prevented altogether by minor treatment, usually as an out-patient. And yes, you should continue on the Pill as it does not interfere with treatment.

An internal examination may be done by a doctor or trained nurse. In the *bimanual examination*—only done usually because of pain symptoms or as part of checking an IUD—the doctor or nurse uses both hands, the left hand on the abdomen and two gloved fingers of the right hand inside the vagina. By applying gentle pressure between both hands, based on previous training and experience, they can then check the shape, size, and normality of the reproductive organs. The other part of the examination is with an instrument called a *speculum*, which enables the doctor or nurse to see inside. The speculum is designed to open out a little so that the walls of the vagina and the entrance to the uterus (the cervix) can be examined. Some women like to put the speculum in for themselves, so you have the choice to ask about that, if you wish. Using a flat wooden or plastic spatula the doctor then wipes some loose cells from the cervix. These cells are transferred to a glass slide or into some special liquid and sent to the laboratory to check that they are normal. This examination, usually taking much less than 5 minutes, is all there is to the well-known cervical smear or 'Pap smear' test.

The speculum may also be used if swabs need to be taken and sent to the laboratory, particularly if you have symptoms that suggest you might have an STI such as chlamydia. If you have recently been with a different sexual partner *or* are afraid your partner may have, because this infection usually causes no symptoms and other STIs might also be present, it is best to have a full check at a GUM or sexual health clinic. Many clinics now offer self-testing for STIs, where you take your own vaginal swab.

You might like to go away and think about your choice of contraceptive. Once you have decided, you should next be given a user-friendly explanatory leaflet—that produced by the FPA still being the best—along with detailed advice about how to use the method and what symptoms need to be promptly reported. If you've chosen the pill, you'll usually be given 3 months' supply at first, to see how it suits you.

You should return for a check-up as instructed, to check blood pressure and any history of headaches, and you will be given further supplies at that time. If you need special supervision because of slightly raised blood pressure or a similar medical reason, you may be asked to come back for the first follow-up sooner than 3 months.

What if I am under age?

If you are under a certain age (16 in Britain, with potentially more enforcement under 13), in many countries your partner will be breaking the law if you have intercourse. Plenty of couples do this, and the law will not lead to any prosecution if there is what it calls 'mutually agreed sexual activity within normal adolescent behaviour, where there is no evidence of exploitation'. But there is a lot more to consider and you should feel under no pressure to have sex until you are ready. Being able to say 'let's wait' could save a lot of worry, and some very real risks: emotional trauma as well as STIs and pregnancy (see Postscript).

If you are already having intercourse under age, know the problems and the risks involved, but feel that it is right for you, you will find that most healthcare providers are prepared to prescribe you the pill—without moralizing. If you have not already done so, they will strongly encourage you to tell at least one of your parents, or some other trusted person like an aunt or older sister. The law recommends but does not enforce this—and actually you could be agreeably surprised by how helpful they turn out to be.

I am under age . . . will they insist on telling my parents?

No. They will recommend to you that *you* involve a parent, but no pressure. Their duty of care and complete confidentiality is just the same as for adults. The slogan is 'Here to listen not to tell!'

It is okay for you to be given the pill even without the definite consent of a parent, if it is the medical judgement of the doctor or nurse that this is in your best interests, and without it your physical or mental health might suffer through the even greater problem of an unwanted pregnancy. Above all they absolutely must keep your confidence: the law says you have the same right to confidentiality as any other (older) person.

Many family doctor services are very welcoming, but if not you will find Brook clinics or the many equivalent young people's clinics in most areas particularly helpful, as they specialize in providing 100 per cent confidential help for teenagers in all sex and contraception matters. They also provide excellent leaflets about sexual health, confidentiality, and talking to doctors.

Counselling and follow-up visits

Counselling for contraception includes an assessment of your personal risks and benefits for the pill, and provides you with the opportunity to ask questions (Box 10.1). Never hesitate to return to whoever prescribed your pills, immediately if necessary, or certainly sooner than your next routine visit, if you ever have doubts or anxieties about using the pill, or about any effect it seems to be having on you.

Box 10.1 Counselling and follow-up

1. If you have a condition that means it is too risky for you to take the pill, you should not go away empty-handed! There are numerous new choices now. Usually *all* of them are options when the pill is contraindicated, since it is primarily the oestrogen that must be avoided. But note that some new ways of taking *both* hormones (rings and patches) also contain oestrogen and so would still be avoided.

2. The first return visit is commonly after 3 months, sooner if special factors apply.

3. All pill users should be monitored to check:
   - Blood pressure.
   - Pattern of headaches, especially migraines.
   - Any symptoms that bother you.
   - Any new illnesses or medicines prescribed.

4. When settled on the pill, healthy women without any risk factors can be seen annually.

5. Some medical or lifestyle conditions mean that the pill should be monitored more carefully (see Chapter 9). This may mean:
   - Being seen at the clinic or surgery more often than usual.
   - Being told if there is anything special to look out for (e.g. changes in migraine) so as to return earlier if necessary.
   - Having special tests done.
   - Being ready to switch to another method of contraception should some current disease worsen or a new risk factor appear—such as migraine with aura or newly raised blood pressure.

If I lose my COCs half way through a packet and my friend has a spare packet of a different brand, is it safe to take them?

This could be a very muddled situation if either yours or hers are phasic pills. Even if they are of the fixed-dose type, it is *not* recommended. However, if there seems no alternative, perhaps when you are away for a weekend, then you should certainly check that the pill is on an equivalent rung of the ladders of Figure 16.1. If it is higher, protection will be maintained, but if it is lower, then protection may be reduced and you should preferably follow the 7-day loss-of-protection rule, using condoms as well as taking the new pills (Chapter 16).

What do I do when I want to get pregnant?

Most family-planning clinics do not deal solely with contraception but can also give you some advice about how to maximize your chances of having a safe, planned pregnancy. They can also check if you need a rubella vaccination. Although rubella is a mild illness in the mother, it can very seriously damage a developing baby during pregnancy. If you plan to have a baby at any time and there is the least doubt about whether you were vaccinated against it as a child, it is sensible to have your immunity to rubella checked at the clinic. Do not rely on a history of German measles in the past: this is often wrong, as other infections can imitate it. If you are not immune, the vaccination is not painful and it is well worth having.

11

How do I start the pill?

➜ Key points

◆ The pill is usually started on the first day of a normal period, which gives immediate contraceptive protection.

◆ If there is no risk of pregnancy, the pill can be started any time during the cycle.

◆ If starting on day 3 or later, additional contraception such as condom should be used for the first 7 days of pill taking.

If you are having normal periods up to the time of starting the pill, there are several different ways to start.

Starting on the first day of the period

This is the routine method in the UK. If, in the first cycle only of pill taking, you start the tablets on the very first day of the period, egg release is effectively prevented even among women with short cycles. Starting the pill without extra contraceptive precautions is absolutely fine up to day 2 of the cycle. This is being a little more cautious than WHO or the FPA, who advise that no additional contraception is necessary for starts up to day 5.

Choose a pill from the section on the packet marked with that day of the week and press the plastic bubble so as to remove it from the foil on the reverse side. Then take a pill each day for 21 days. After a 7-day break you then start taking pills again on the eighth day: and from then on in each 4 weeks you follow the regular routine of 21 days of pill taking followed by a 7-day break. Avoid a common mistake, which is to start each new packet on the first day of the period. This can cause a pregnancy if the 'period' happens to come on late.

BTB, which is bleeding on days when you are taking tablets, is common in the first few months (Fig. 11.1) but usually settles by the time the third packet of pills is started.

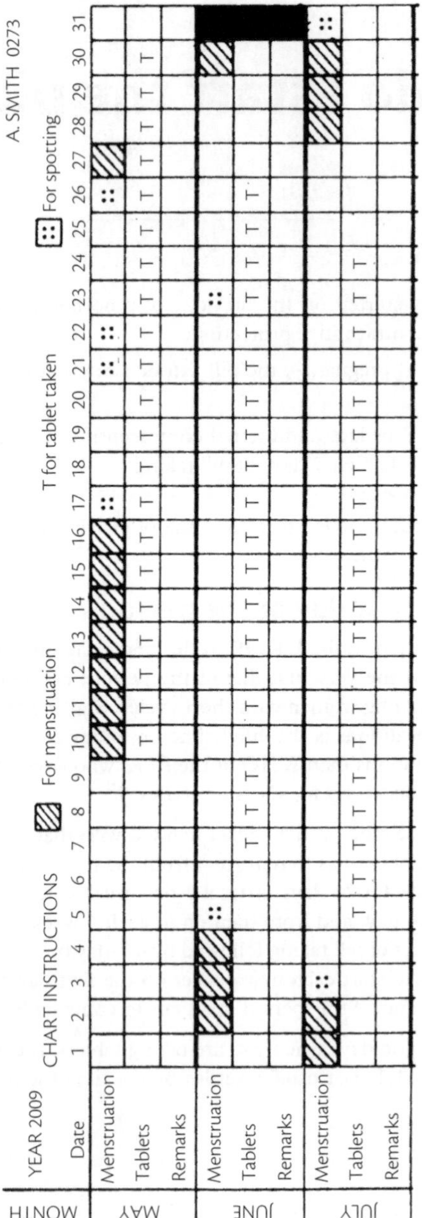

Figure 11.1 Diary card: first-day start of the pill.

Note: some expected extra days of spotting and bleeding occur in the first cycle, which is also short (about 24 days).

It is important to realize that your first hormone withdrawal bleed on the pill will come on sooner than usual. This is because you will be taking your 21st tablet only 21 days after the start of the previous period. As usual on the pill, your 'period'/hormone withdrawal bleeding follows only a day or two after that. Thus the very first pill cycle will tend to be only about 23 days long, but this matters not at all. The next packet is started as usual after 7 days whether or not a 'period' happens and however long it lasts.

Starting on the fifth day of the period

This method is not often used now. You take the first pill on the fifth day of your period, whether your bleeding has stopped or not. The snag of this system is that some women frequently—and others 'out of the blue'—can have short menstrual cycles. There is then the small risk that there may already at this stage in the cycle be a follicle ripening. This could be producing so much natural oestrogen that the pill may be unable to stop the surge of LH from the pituitary, which leads to release of an egg (see Chapter 2). We recommend that until the seventh pill of the first course has been taken you should use an effective alternative method of contraception as well, such as the condom.

'Sunday start'

Starting on the first Sunday after your period starts, with extra precautions (just in the first cycle) right through until you have taken the first 7 days of *active* tablets, is usual in the USA and some countries. An advantage is that the 21st or last pill of that and of each subsequent pack—or the last *active* pill if ED ('every day') packs are being used—will be on a Saturday. The withdrawal bleed will then begin on a weekday, probably the Monday, so no bleeding at weekends! But even without a Sunday start, it is still possible to avoid weekend periods, just by having a shortening (*not* lengthening) of the pill-free interval for one cycle (see 'Lisa' in Chapter 12).

'Quick start'

If you have not had any sex at all since your last period began, or if you are 100 per cent confident that no sperm escaped when condoms were used, you could also start the pill on any day of your cycle, with condoms as well for at least the next 7 days. If the risk of having conceived before the pill-start is acceptably low, the only other likely problem is irregular bleeding—which will nearly always settle in the first two to three cycles.

Quick start of the pill may also be acceptable sometimes after emergency hormonal contraception, rather than, as would be more usual (and officially licensed) waiting till the first or second day of the next period.

Sally wanted to start the pill as she was about to go on holiday with her boyfriend, who she usually only managed to see intermittently. She knew that she had to wait until the first day of her period to start the pill. Unfortunately, her period was due to start halfway through the holiday. She was delighted to find that since she had not had sex since her last period she could start the pill straightaway. Not only would it be effective by the time she went on holiday, she should avoid a period while she was away.

Starting phasic pills

With phasic pills, treatment starts as usual on the first day of your period, with no extra precautions. Always take the pill phases in the correct order! Logynon ED® contains 21 small active pills in three rows (six light brown, five white, and ten ochre-coloured), then seven larger white inactive tablets. It has a special starting system (Box 11.1), very like that for Microgynon ED® and Femodene ED® and explained in the PIL leaflet with each pack.

Box 11.1 How to start Logynon ED®

◆ The first Logynon ED® pill in the foil pack is marked 'start'.

◆ There is also a set of seven self-adhesive strips, each starting with a different day of the week. Peel off the strip that starts with your starting day. For instance, if your period starts on a Wednesday, use the one that starts with 'Wed'.

◆ Stick the strip along the top of the foil pack so that the first day is above the pill marked 'start'. You will now see on which day to take each tablet and will have contraceptive protection at once.

◆ After you have taken all 28 daily pills (during the inactive, larger white ones you will have your 'period'): fix a new sticky strip to the next pack and take the pill marked 'start', on your same start day.

If transferring from another pill higher up a ladder, or if you are in any doubt about the relative strength of your new pill, it is best to follow the rules in Chapter 15, i.e. immediate transfer from the last pill of the old packet to the first of the phasic pill, with no need for extra precautions.

Starting after a recent pregnancy

There is no need to wait for your first period after a baby. Indeed to do so may well mean you conceive with the very first egg you release after the previous birth! Even if you do not breastfeed, egg release does not happen earlier than about 4 weeks after delivery. So, if you are *bottle-feeding,* you start taking the pill *from the 21st day* after the birth (no extra precautions needed). Twenty-one days later, when you finish the first packet, you should see the first withdrawal bleed.

It is better not to start earlier, as this might increase the small risk of thrombosis (clotting) in a vein of the legs that persists for a couple of weeks after giving birth. But starting later is a choice, so long as another method such as condoms is used carefully up until starting the pill and until seven daily pills have been taken. If you get unexpected bleeding, as heavy as a period, and especially if it is painful, in the first weeks after any pregnancy has ended, it could mean that part of the placenta remains behind, in the uterus. So see your doctor or one of the doctors at the hospital *without delay.*

How soon after starting am I protected against pregnancy?

Immediately, provided that contraception is started 21 days after a full-term baby; or if started the day after a miscarriage or termination of pregnancy; or on day 1—or even up to day 3—of the menstrual cycle. Otherwise, for maximum reliability alternative precautions such as the condom should be used until seven tablets have been taken.

Starting after another hormonal method

Generally you will be recommended to start the pill on the same day as stopping the old method. Removal of the IUD or IUS is also often delayed until the pill has been safely started, meaning again a bit of 'overlap'.

If in doubt, e.g. if you have not been seeing any kind of bleeding or a proper cycle with your last method, bring a urine specimen with you and discuss how to start with your doctor or nurse.

12

How do I take the pill?

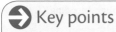 Key points

◆ The pill is usually taken daily, for 21–24 days out of every 28.

◆ Sex during the pill break is only protected if a new pill pack is started on time.

◆ Women who have unwanted symptoms only during the pill-free week, or who would benefit from enhanced contraceptive efficacy, should consider either tricycling (three or four packets back-to-back) or taking the pill continuously 365/365.

Regular pill taking

If the pill is the method for you, regularity is vital. It can be taken morning, noon, or night as long as it is at a roughly constant time, preferably within an hour or two.

Take your pill at least 4 hours before or after you drink any grapefruit juice, as this can raise the blood levels of oestrogen.

A useful trick is to set a regular daily alarm on your mobile. There is now estimated to be 24 hours' leeway in pill taking for pregnancy prevention. This means that you can easily catch up if you forget overnight, for example: but it is decidedly unwise to make a habit of this. The reason for being consistent is that, after each pill is absorbed, your liver and kidneys, working in combination, are continually eliminating the hormones of the pill from your body. So a gap of more than the usual 24 hours between tablets certainly increases the chance of BTB due to too little pill support to the womb's lining. More importantly, if you are late in taking or miss out the first pill(s) of the *next* pack, you will risk breakthrough egg release and pregnancy—since this prolongs the time when your body has anyway just had a week's rest from the pill's effects.

The risk of pregnancy if pills are forgotten is also greater if you are on a pill containing 20 mcg or less of EE, or if you are being treated with any drug which might interfere with the pill's actions (see Chapter 15).

Does crossing time zones mean I have to change the time I take the pill?

Suppose you fly from Auckland to London and normally take your pill at bedtime. If you then switch to taking it at the London bedtime you would have a 36-hour interval between tablets. This is actually OK and you are still contraceptively safe, as you are only 12 hours late from your usual pill-taking time. *But* don't make it longer and get back to taking it regularly at bedtime... You might get some irregular or breakthrough bleeding (BTB) for a couple of days.

If the journey was eastbound, taking that day's pill at the correct local time will shorten the real pill-taking interval and this is always contraceptively safer.

How many days a month do I take the pill for?

When the pill was first available on prescription in 1962, the standard system was the 21/7 system—21 days of pill taking followed by a 7-day break. As the doses of hormones in the pill have got lower, coupled with the realization that there is no clear-cut necessity for a 'pill-free' week, other patterns of pill taking have been developed.

21/7 system

The traditional system is the one in which you take one pill daily—morning, evening, or any other regular time that you find easy to remember—for 21 days, followed by a 7-day break taking nothing at all. There are also some ED brands available with 28 tablets in each packet, of which seven are dummies or 'blanks'. ED pills are taken consecutively, one packet after another so are particularly good for helping the user not to make the worst kind of pill-taking mistake: which is being *late in restarting* pill taking after that regular 7-day break from the pill's contraceptive effects.

Is it safe to have sex on the during the 7- day break?

Yes: *but only* if no pills have been missed (or not absorbed) towards the end of the previous pill packet, and you do in fact start another packet on time after the pill-free week. The safety of this time depends on the *next packet* (or patch or ring) as much as on the one that came before. This vital need to restart on time after those 7 days without the contraception is something just as true of EVRA® and NuvaRing® as well!

24/4 system

The 7-day break from the pill is the real 'Achilles' heel' of contraception. Any break from the pill allows for ovaries to 'wake-up' with the potential for contraceptive failure. This is a particular concern with the ultra-low-dose pills. Hence, Yaz® which has only 4 days of placebo tablets following 24 days of pill-taking.

In the USA, the FDA have also approved Loestrin 24 Fe® containing 24 days of active hormones followed by 4 days of ferrous fumate (iron) tablets instead of placebo.

Tricycle system

Even with a shortened hormone-free interval to improve contraceptive efficacy, pill breaks can still be problematic for some women who experience headaches, fatigue, pelvic cramps, irritability, mood swings and other symptoms at this time. Hence the *3-monthly* or '*tricycle' system* (Fig. 12.1).

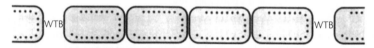

Figure 12.1 Tricycling (using four packs).
Note: they must be monophasic packs. The duration of the pill-free interval may also be shortened. WTB, withdrawal bleeding.

In this, four packs are taken in succession—therefore a pill every day for up to 84 days—followed by a break during which the 'period' normally occurs. As explained in Chapter 1, pill 'periods' are in fact 'hormone withdrawal bleeds', created artificially by the taking of a seven-day break. So there is no particular reason why they should not happen every 13 weeks, with the four-packs-in-a-row system, instead of every four weeks. Once this has been explained, many find this four-per-year routine perfectly acceptable or even preferable. In the US, an 84/7 pill is called Seasonale® since the user only bleeds once a season—summer, autumn, winter, and spring!

As shown in Box 12.1, there are some special reasons why the doctor may recommend this even without your particular preference.

If you get symptoms in the pill-free week, you may not like even four breaks a year. To partly address this problem, Seasonique®, a sister pill to Seasonale®, was approved by the FDA in 2006. Instead of 7 days of dummy pills, 84 days of active pill are followed by 7 days of tablets containing 10 mcg of EE. These tablets contain one-third of the dose of EE used in the rest of the cycle, and no progestogen. This very low dose of oestrogen helps to eliminate symptoms that may occur with complete hormone withdrawal.

Box 12.1 Reasons for tricycling of the pill

1. Personal choice.

2. If headaches or other symptoms are a problem in the pill-free week. Tricycling means, at most, five bad headaches a year instead of 13.

3. If the 'periods' themselves are bad.

4. To treat premenstrual syndrome (PMS).

5. To manage epilepsy and other conditions treated with drugs that interact with the pill.

6. To treat endometriosis.

7. If there has been previous failure of the pill, leading to pregnancy.

But the biggest problem is annoying bleeding at the wrong times, especially towards the end of the sequence of packs: you may then be advised to take a few days break from tablet taking and restart. Thereafter fewer packs in a row—e.g. 'bi-cycling'—might work better for you.

Note that the tricycle system of pill taking is of course completely different from triphasic pills. Indeed it does not work satisfactorily with any phasic pills: the more common single-phase (monophasic) brands need to be used.

365/365 continuous-dose system

Of course, any problems with the hormone-free interval can be avoided completely if the pill is taken continuously, without a break. This also means that women can avoid having 'periods', rather than the usual 13 a year. In May 2007, the FDA approved Lybrel®, a product continuing low-dose combination pills taken every day. Lybrel® comes in a 28-day pack with each pill containing just 20 mcg of EE and 90 mcg of LNG. As with tricycling, irregular spotting and bleeding are the main problem that can occur, but usually diminish over time. Lybrel® is not available in the UK, but doctor's sometimes recommended low-dose 21-day pills, taken back-to-back, without a break. Continuous Loestrin 20® seems more likely to achieve no bleeding at all than other currently available brands. One good thing with 20mcg products is that the total dose per year is only 7300 mcg—compared with 8190 mcg for a 30 mcg pill taken 21/7.

Postponing or changing the timing of 'periods'

Even if you regularly use the system of three weeks on, one week off, one advantage of the pill is that you always have the option of postponing your 'period'. When planning for your holidays, for example, this can be done either by taking extra pills from a spare packet, or more simply by just taking two or three packets in succession.

Lisa's boyfriend is at a different university and they can only meet at weekends. The pill suits her and gives her regular bleeds but (just because her first period when she started the pill 5 years ago happened to start on a Thursday) she has been stopping each pack on Wednesdays. Therefore, when she bleeds it is always from Friday to Monday. Now, as a one-off, she stops as usual on the Wednesday but starts again with an active pill on the next Sunday: sorted!

Phasic pills

With a phasic pill (except Synphase®, whose third phase is identical to the first) the switch from the higher progestogen dose of the last phase to the low dose of the first phase tends to cause withdrawal bleeding. So there are two options (Fig. 12.2):

♦ *Take extra pills from the last phase of a different packet.* This will give a maximum of 10 days' postponement with Trinordiol®/Logynon®, for example, using the yellow tablets; or 7 days using the third phase of Trinovum® (which can conveniently be snapped off);

♦ *Interpose a packet of the next higher brand up the same ladder in Fig. 16.1.* You should make an 'instant' switch from the phasic pill to the fixed-dose

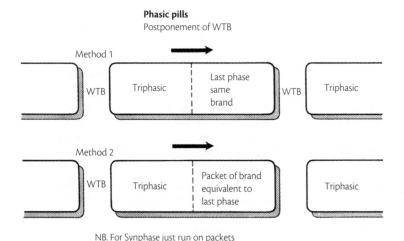

Phasic pills
Postponement of WTB

NB. For Synphase just run on packets

Figure 12.2 Two possible methods for short-term postponement of withdrawal bleeding (WTB) by women using phasic pills.
Note: the brand 'equivalent to the last phase' will be a monophasic pill with a (near-) identical formulation, e.g. Microgynon®/Ovranette® in the case of the triphasic levonorgestrel pills Logynon®/Trinordiol®. See Table 16.1.

brand—i.e. no days without pill taking till the end of a 42-tablet sequence. This should give at least 6 weeks free of bleeding.

> Susie wanted to avoid a 'period' while she was on holiday. Her last Trinordiol® pill was on a Monday. She took the first tablet (marked Tuesday) from a Microgynon 30® packet. Three weeks later she took the last Microgynon® on her usual finishing day, a Monday. She had her 'period' during the 7-day break and then started Trinordiol®, as usual taking the Tuesday tablet from the first section of another Trinordiol® packet.

Stopping the pill

At what age should I stop the pill?

Healthy non-smokers with a normal BMI may if they so choose take one of the lowest-dose pills until age 51. You should stop the pill at 35 if you have any risk factors, or if you smoke 15 or more a day (although many doctors feel uncomfortable about any smoking in a woman over 35 on the pill).

Coming off the pill (routinely)

Although I had very regular 'periods' on the pill I stopped taking it some months ago and have still not had a period. What does this mean?

In about 1–2 per cent of women the first period is very much delayed. It means that your natural menstrual cycle, with egg release and periods, has not yet been restored. It is sensible to take medical advice—but not until 6 months have gone by. Then a few tests are important, to check that your pituitary gland and ovaries are in good working order, albeit currently 'resting'.

Two-thirds of women have their first period by 6 weeks after their last pill 'period'. If you do not get your period by then, do a pregnancy test on a small amount of your first urine of the day. Commonly it will be negative and remain so if repeated, until you see your first natural period in due course. But see your doctor or family-planning nurse if you have other symptoms, particularly pain which could (rarely) be from an ectopic. This would happen because of a previously damaged tube, perhaps from a chlamydia infection years earlier that you never knew you had—and the pill would have been stopping you from getting the ectopic (perhaps for many years), just like it stops the more normal kind of pregnancy.

When I stop the pill to take a break for a while, can I assume protection for the next 7 days like in the usual hormone-free break?

Emphatically *not*! The pill only protects against pregnancy during the pill-free break *provided that you start a new pack*! So, unless you want to get pregnant, you need to start a different method of contraception the day after you take your last pill, if not before. If you don't follow this rule, sex during this time is unprotected and you might need the emergency pill. The same approach applies to the patch and ring.

Stopping the pill to have a baby

Women who stop the pill to have a planned baby are still usually advised to use another contraceptive method, such as condoms, until they have had one natural period—which means the one after the 'withdrawal' bleeding which followed the last packet of pills. There are no particular medical concerns about getting pregnant soon after stopping the pill, but it is easier to 'date' the start of the pregnancy from a natural period.

How often should I take a 'break' from the pill?

It's a common myth but there is no good medical reason to recommend the need for a 'break' from the pill. One way of looking at this is: because you take the pill for only three weeks in four, even if you have only been on it for 4 years, you've really only taken it for 3 years, with 52 weeks of short breaks. How many more do you want?

Abnormal measurements on pill treatment, including changed clotting factors, often return towards normal during the 7-day pill-free intervals. Could these breaks actually be important as a time of 'rest' for the system, a time when the body adjusts before the next 3 weeks of pill taking? That is so far only hypothetical.

In practice, many women find out the hard way that their fertility is fine, by stopping the pill just because 'someone said they should have a break'—and getting pregnant! So if you are not ready for a baby, consider staying on the pill, or at least use another effective contraceptive from the day you stop. Note that fertility-awareness methods are unreliable, generally, until after two normal periods have happened.

Intermittent breaks from the pill are a nuisance, are of no proven benefit for health, and also have been known to lead to unplanned pregnancies.

What It Is It Like to Take a Break for a while

Simply ... to take a ...

How often Should I take a ... Break, ...?

13

What if I forget a pill?

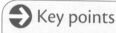 **Key points**

- For the pill to protect against pregnancy, it must be taken regularly and on time.

- Sex in the pill-free week is only protected if a new pack is started on time and the previous pack was taken correctly.

- The most dangerous pills to miss are in the first or last 7 days of a pack. If you miss more than one pill at this time you may need emergency contraception.

Don't panic if you forget to take a pill. This is one of the most common worries that any pill user ever has. It is unlikely that you will become pregnant. However, it is certainly not something to make a habit of it as it is the reason for most pill failures. To be as safe as can be you need to follow some simple recommendations. Firstly, you need to understand that the riskiest time to miss pills is either side of the pill-free interval.

What if I forget to start a new pack after the 7-day pill-free break?

If you have had sex during the pill-free break, you are only protected from pregnancy if you follow three golden rules:

1. You must have been regular in your pill taking throughout the preceding packet.

2. Nothing that might reduce your protection, like vomiting back a tablet, has happened near the end of the previous pack (Chapter 16).

3. Above all, *you do in fact start another packet on the eighth day, on time.*

Research has shown that during the pill-free week, there is a rise in the blood levels of FSH (from the pituitary gland) and oestrogen (from a follicle growing in one of the ovaries, as can be observed with an ultrasound scanner). The rise is more marked in some women (about 20 per cent) than in others. This means that the pituitary and ovaries of these women are, if you like, close to escaping from the suppressing effect of the pill (Chapter 2). Any lengthening of the pill-free time beyond 7 days means a risk that the ovary 'wakes up'. If so, follicle growth and oestrogen production in some women can be high enough to cause a 'surge' of LH and hence egg release from the largest follicle. With egg release comes the risk of pregnancy (Fig. 13.1).

So never make the mistake of starting the next packet late or missing any of the first seven pills in the pack. Contrary to what many think, being late starting even by just 1 day is much more risky than missing, say, three or even four pills in the middle of the pack. This is because the 7-day break from pill taking is a *contraceptive-free* time, during which your ovaries are not getting any effects from the pill.

If you ever make this break longer than 7 days, your ovaries might release an egg early in the following week. And then, of course, if you have had sex during the non-pill-taking days, the sperm might survive long enough to fertilize that egg. But do not worry otherwise; if you *don't* lengthen the pill-free time beyond that critical 7 days, then intercourse is safe on any day of any month. An easy way to remember this is to consider the 7-day slogan (Box 13.1).

Box 13.1 The 7-day slogan

◆ Seven days of pill taking always puts the ovaries to sleep.

◆ Any more tablets taken after the first seven keep the ovaries asleep and inactive.

◆ Up to seven missed pills (as in the pill-free week) is contraceptively safe provided it is immediately followed by the first tablet of a new pack.

◆ More than 7 days since the last pill was taken risks the ovaries 'waking up' (egg release).

An even simpler slogan for the pill take is: 'I MUST NEVER BE A LATE RESTARTER'.

The modern advice for missed pills is therefore based on when, in each week of pill taking, the pills were missed, and is summarized in Figure 2.5 in Chapter 2. Notice that a single missed pill is defined as a whole day late (24 hours).

Where an 'extra method' is recommended, in this figure or (in other chapters) to do with other hormonal methods, the other method must *never* be the rhythm, temperature, or cervical mucus methods. The pill's hormones make these quite unusable. Contraceptive experts do not recommend spermicides for use alone either, and the IUD or IUS is unlikely to be useful for so short a time. So what is usually meant is either abstinence or a (male or female) condom.

The advice here is a bit different from what you read in the FPA leaflet that you may have been given, and probably also the PIL that comes with the pill packet. This is because, in our opinion, there should be one simple set of rules

Every time you miss any one pill (late by up to 24 hours)

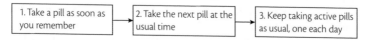

If you miss more than one pill—meaning anything more than 24 hours have passed since the time an active pill should have been taken:

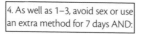

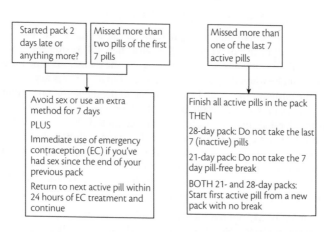

4. As well as 1–3, avoid sex or use an extra method for 7 days AND:

Started pack 2 days late or anything more?	Missed more than two pills of the first 7 pills		Missed more than one of the last 7 active pills

Avoid sex or use an extra method for 7 days
PLUS
Immediate use of emergency contraception (EC) if you've had sex since the end of your previous pack
Return to next active pill within 24 hours of EC treatment and continue

Finish all active pills in the pack
THEN
28-day pack: Do not take the last 7 (inactive) pills
21-day pack: Do not take the 7 day pill-free break
BOTH 21- and 28-day packs: Start first active pill from a new pack with no break

28-day packs: if you miss any of the inactive pills ONLY, return to the right pill or the day before and make sure that you start the new pack on time

Figure 13.1 Advice for missed pills.

Note: NB plural! Missing a single pill for up to 24 hours means only actions 1→3 at the top of the figure.

*For what to do if more than 4 are missed in days 8–21, see text.

**Even with triphasic pills, you should go straight to (the first phase of) the same brand. You may bleed a bit but you will still strengthen your contraception.

***28-pill or ED packs such as Microgynon-ED* can be very helpful, to minimize the risk of being a 'late restarter' of active pills, after the 7-day 'contraception-losing' time.

that gives the contraceptively safest advice, whichever strength of pill is used. Beware, sometimes in some countries the manufacturer's advice has actually been contraceptively unsafe.

Missing pills at the beginning of a packet

The first obvious way a woman might accidentally lengthen the pill-free time could be by being late restarting after the pill break, or forgetting one or more pills in the first week of a packet. Either will significantly lengthen the time without the pill's contraceptive actions. In fact, going away for a weekend or longer without one's pills, having sex while away, and then starting the next packet late (something a lot of people don't even reckon as 'missing pills') is a well-known cause of unplanned pregnancy. That is one reason to consider use of 28-day ED pill packaging.

The advice in Figure 13.1 should protect you if you completely miss one or more pills early in a packet but you must also not rely solely on the pill method, for 7 days from the moment you discover the problem.

Missing pills at the end of a packet

Another way a woman might lengthen the pill-free time would be by missing pills at the *end* of the previous packet, and then still taking the usual 7-day break. In this case if you take no special action the dangerous time for conceiving would not be when the pills were forgotten, but *over a week later* when—once again—the pituitary and ovary have been 'let off the hook' for longer than usual. In fact, pregnancy could result from intercourse during or after the (falsely reassuring) 'period' that comes *after* the missed pills! This is because that bleeding is not truly a period, being caused only by the withdrawal of the artificial hormones. It has no connection with what is happening at the ovary. The egg could be released around the end of the pill-free time *whenever it has been made longer than usual—unless you act*. So, the advice is: get back to pill taking and miss out the next active pill-free days.

This means you may not have a period until the end of two packs in a row, but this does you no harm. Nor does it matter, whenever pills have been missed, if for a while you see some BTB on subsequent tablet-taking days.

Missing pills in the middle of a packet

Contrary to what most pill takers—and some doctors—think, the middle of a packet is the least dangerous time to miss tablets. Egg release and pregnancy are very unlikely because the pills are missed after the pituitary and ovary have been 'put to sleep' by that 'magic minimum' of 7 days of pill taking (see Box 13.1). The advice to use condoms for 7 days (Fig. 13.1) is so ultra-cautious that if you did not do so, you would *not* need emergency contraception unless perhaps, you had missed more than 4 pills!

Missing/forgetting a succession of pills

Should you ask for emergency (post-coital) contraception? *Emergency contraception* (see Chapter 18) is already advised in Figure 13.1 for the worst situation, *where you are 2 days late or anything more in restarting after the break, or have missed two or more tablets out of the first seven,* and you also had intercourse since the end of the previous packet. It is also usually given, just to be on the safe side, if more than four pills in a row have been missed in the middle week.

But however many pills were missed in the third week (tablets 15–21), running straight on to the next pack should always be enough. It is only if you don't run on that emergency contraception would be needed: since the total pill-free time would be more than 7 days.

What about triphasic pills?

The rules are the same. If you have missed pills at the end of a packet and therefore follow the advice and switch straight to the very low dose of the first phase, you are a bit more liable to get a bleed than on a monophasic pill. But contraception will still be improved with either pill type. If postponing bleeding more than restoring contraception is your main concern, and a phasic pill is involved, see Chapter 12.

14

What else can make the pill less effective?

> ### → Key points
>
> ◆ The effectiveness of the pill is reduced by anything that interferes with the normal absorption or metabolism of the pill hormones.
>
> ◆ This includes vomiting within 2 hours of pill taking and certain drugs.

This chapter discusses some of the more common medical reasons why pills can fail. But don't forget that missed pills are the most common reason for 'pill' pregnancies. If you miss any pills, especially at the start of a new packet, follow the advice in Chapter 13.

Stomach upsets

You can 'miss' pills by severe vomiting: it means the same for the body as forgetting to take pills. The risks of breakthrough egg release and BTB are increased in just the same way.

The advice to be followed is as for missed pills (see Chapter 13), based on when in the packet the vomiting occurred and the number of pills that were not kept down.

If any single episode of vomiting was more than 2 hours after pill taking, according to the WHO no action is required at all, as by then the pill would have passed beyond your stomach. However, if you vomit back a correctly timed pill after less than 2 hours, you should take another as soon as you feel you will keep it down. If that one stays down and was taken within a day (less than 24 hours) of the vomited tablet then, again, you can continue to rely on the pill as your method. Should your stomach reject a second or even more pills, you should get back to taking tablets as soon as you are able to keep them down, and follow the advice in Box 14.1 and Chapter 13.

Box 14.1 How many pills have you vomited?

◆ More than four pills of any of the pills in the middle week, days 8–14: no special action.

◆ Any pills from days 15–21: go straight on to your next pack: no further action.

◆ Two or more tablets during days 1–7 of new pack:

· take emergency contraception *and*

· abstain or use condoms until seven tablets have been taken (without being vomited back!).

If you have lost pills through vomiting, extra ones should ideally be taken from a separate packet or, in an emergency, from the end of the current packet (making sure you get a new supply so that you don't lengthen the *next* pill-free interval). This means that you can continue taking the right pill for each day of the week. If you are using a phasic pill, ensure that the replacement pill is the same colour.

Diarrhoea alone (without vomiting) has to be 'as bad as cholera' to interfere with the absorption of the pill. If it is like that, which means like water and every few minutes, follow the advice just given for a bad attack of vomiting. Otherwise just keep taking your tablets. Note that with EVRA® and NuvaRing®, since they do not enter via the stomach at all, there's no problem here!

The effect of other medicines on the pill

To be effective, the pill must be absorbed, be transported in the blood, perform its actions, and then be eliminated from the body. A number of other drugs can interfere with some of these complex processes. Such interference (interaction) can lower the blood levels of the pill hormones and so lead to the risk of egg release and therefore pregnancy (see Box 14.2).

This weakening contraception effect can be caused in various ways. The most important is when enzyme inducers are prescribed. These medicines, in addition to their main effect, have a simulating action on special liver enzymes that normally inactivate pill hormones before they leave the body via the bowels and in the urine. So more inactivation means weaker contraception.

Secondly, some *antibiotics* are able, when they reach the large bowel, to kill certain 'friendly' bacteria which normally help to keep up the blood levels of the pill's oestrogen, so allowing the bowel to reabsorb some of this (which is otherwise on its way out of the body). These antibiotics might therefore lower the oestrogen levels. Though this weakens contraception in only a very small number of women, no one knows which women are at risk. So in UK practice

Box 14.2 Important drugs which are suspected of interfering with the pill, causing BTB and increased risk of pregnancy (see text)

Drugs to treat epilepsy

- Phenobarbital (Luminal®) and other barbiturates.
- Phenytoin (Epanutin®).
- Primidone (Mysoline®).
- Carbamazepine (Tegretol®) and oxcarbazepine (Trileptal®).
- Topiramate (Topamax®).
- Modafinil (Provigil®)—used to treat excessive sleepiness.

Note: Other drugs for epilepsy do not interfere at all, including sodium valproate (Epilim®), clonazepam (Rivotril®), lamotrigine (Lamictal®), and vigabatrin (Sabril®). If you are taking lamotrigine and start the pill, patch, or ring, discuss this with whoever manages your epilepsy treatment as you may need a higher dose of lamotrigine to control your attacks.

Drugs to treat infections

- Rifampicin (Rimactane®) and rifabutin (Mycobutin®) used in the treatment of tuberculosis and some other infections.
- Griseofulvin (Grisovin®)—antifungal.

Miscellaneous enzyme-inducing drugs

- Some anti-retroviral drugs used to treat HIV/AIDS (details at http://www.hiv-drug interactions.org).
- St John's Wort ('Nature's Prozac')—its potency as sold is so variable that the CSM advises it is not used along with the pill.

Note: All the above are enzyme inducers (see text).

There is a possibility that other antibiotics, such as amoxicillin (Amoxil®) and tetracyclines (note that doxycycline is also an anti-malarial), may also have a weakening effect on the pill, but much less than any of the above and only for a limited time (see text). There is no concern if you take erythromycin (Erythrocin®), co-trimoxazole (Septrin®), or metronidazole (Flagyl®), which seem to enhance the pill's effects by inhibiting the liver's actions.

Note: this is not a complete list. Other drug interactions remain to be clarified. Several here have been deliberately omitted because so far there is too little evidence that, in practice, they cause any problem for pill users. Except for doxycycline, which is a tetracycline (see above), anti-malarial drugs are OK.

it is still considered safest to assume all women taking these antibiotics might be affected.

> If you are in doubt about whether or not any medicines you are taking might interfere with the pill:
>
> 1. Tell the person who prescribes you the pill about all other medicines you are taking.
> 2. Inform any other doctor about to prescribe you *any treatment* that you use the pill. For safety, ask them specifically about any effect on the pill.

If you are put on a relevant medicine, especially one from Box 15.2, use another contraceptive method such as the condom throughout the treatment, and when it finishes continue extra precautions for seven more days; if you are now in the last week of a pack, run on to the next packet without a break.

Long-term antibiotics: treatment for at least 2 weeks

This applies to relevant broad-spectrum antibiotics *(not rifampicin, rifabutin, or griseofulvin)*. The special system mentioned above, which in some women may help to keep oestrogen blood levels up, depends on friendly bacteria in the bowel which are killed by the antibiotic. These become resistant to the antibiotic after about 2 weeks, and so they come back in large enough numbers to do their good work. This is why extra precautions are unnecessary if you are already taking long-term, low-dose tetracycline antibiotics when starting the pill. The only time they are recommended is the other way around, if the antibiotic is started in a current pill taker. This would be during all the treatment days and for 1 week thereafter, to a maximum of 3 weeks (i.e. 2 weeks plus one for contraceptive safety). If the last week of a pill pack is involved, skip the next contraception-free interval.

> Lucy takes the combined pill. She is going abroad and is starting doxy-cyline to protect against malaria. She will continue to take her pill, using condoms only for the first 3 weeks of treatment, and running two pill-packs together to skip the pill-free break.

> Amy is on long-term tetracycline for acne and wants to take the pill. She does not need to use any additional contraception if she starts the pill on the first day of her period.

Enzyme inducers

The drugs concerned are chiefly treatments for tuberculosis or epilepsy. If you are taking such drugs, usually long-term, you should first consider using another method of contraception altogether—ideally an intrauterine method or injection (see Chapter 3).

After discussion, though, you may be able to continue to take the pill in a special way (Box 14.3) which as it is not how the pill is licensed will have to be *authorized by a doctor* as a so-called 'named patient use'.

Box 14.3 COC and enzyme inducers

◆ Use two tablets totalling 50–60 mcg of the oestrogen, making a higher-dose pill to compensate for the lowered blood levels caused by the enzyme inducer.

◆ Take fewer 'contraceptively dangerous' breaks than usual between pill packets, i.e. use the tricycling scheme.

◆ The break after each run of four packets should be additionally shortened to 4 days.

◆ Consider a continuous pill, with no breaks.

Isn't it dangerous to take high doses (two pills) every day?

For women taking enzyme-inducing drugs, it is still the same for the body as taking one pill. The extra hormones are being got rid of faster by the medication speeding up the liver's metabolism. This leaves only the same amount in the system as other pill takers would get from one pill a day. It's a bit like *climbing up a down escalator* to stay in the same place.

Watch out for bleeding on tablet-taking days. This bleeding coming on for the first time after starting another drug can be the early warning sign of too low a blood level of the pill's hormones. Sometimes BTB is just a consequence of the tricycling itself, happening late in a sequence of packs. Either way the BTB symptom should always be discussed promptly with whoever prescribes you the pill.

If you are on an enzyme-inducing drug and a higher-dose pill, be careful if you stop the enzyme inducer. You should normally stay on the higher dose of contraception or use added contraception with condoms for 1 month, before going back to the planned single-tablet dose alone. The reason is that for a considerable time after the inducer drug is stopped, the liver goes on being more efficient than usual at getting rid of the pill's hormones.

The effect of the pill on other drugs

The opposite kind of interference is also possible, in which the pill alters the blood levels of another drug.

◆ Ciclosporin, used after transplant surgery, is one drug for which the pill can increase blood levels, which may need to be measured to avoid overdosing.

◆ Lamotrigine, used in the treatment of epilepsy, can have its blood levels lowered by the pill. Therefore, if someone already taking this drug starts the pill, their epilepsy may be less well controlled.

As a pill taker, the main thing is that *if in doubt,* ask if the other drug matters, either way. Fortunately, very few actually make an important difference to treatment.

Over-the-counter, herbal, and illegal drugs

Except for St John's Wort, the good news is that none of the medicines available over the counter in the UK seems to weaken the pill's contraceptive effects. And so-called 'recreational' or illegal drugs (and alcohol) have loads of other problems, but none of them are known to cause the pill to fail this way—though all of them may make the user so spaced-out she fails to take the pill properly!

Change of pills from a higher- to a lower-dose variety

This matter of the different brands of pills will make more sense when you have read Chapter 17. However, the question of changing to a lower-dose pill needs to be considered here, as this is another time when there could be some loss of contraceptive protection. At the changeover time, the steady suppression by the pill of the woman's natural hormones from her pituitary and ovary is reduced, just enough perhaps to allow breakthrough egg release 'on the rebound'. However, once she is safely established on the new ultra-low-dose pill, she is effectively protected against pregnancy. The extra pregnancy risk is only at the time of the changeover and is believed to be small: indeed some experts question if it is real at all. It can be virtually eliminated by taking extra precautions during the first seven pills, if there is the usual gap between packets. More simply, the recommended method is to *start the new lower-dose variety the very next day after finishing the current higher-dose packet.*

If you follow this system, you may have bleeding like a pill 'period' during the first 7 days of tablet taking from your new low-dose packet. Or you may have no bleeding at all until after the end of that new packet. Either is quite normal, and your protection against pregnancy is maintained throughout.

Of course this problem never arises when moving to a definitely higher-dose pill, which can be done after the usual 7-day break. If you are ever left in doubt about what your new pill is, act as though it is lower dose.

For the rules about changing from a combined (ordinary) pill (COC) to a progestogen-only variety (POP) or back again, see Chapter 17.

15

What if I get side-effects?

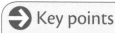 Key points

- So-called 'minor' side-effects such as breakthrough bleeding, nausea, and breast tenderness are common and do not require early review unless troublesome or cause concern.

- Serious side-effects are rare but should be reviewed by a doctor as soon as possible and may mean that the pill should be stopped immediately.

If I get a bad side-effect, can I stop the pill in the middle of a packet/cycle?

Yes, though if you are having sex it must be beyond day 7, because of the rule that '7 days of pill-taking puts the ovaries to sleep' reliably. Even then, with the pill it is best to complete the sequence, otherwise you will get a bleed prematurely. But if the reason for stopping is one of the possibly serious symptoms mentioned below you should still be able to avoid a pregnancy if you transfer *immediately* to using another method, such as the condom.

Non-serious side-effects

Changes in bleeding patterns are probably the most frequently reported side-effects of the pill, particularly when the pill is first started. Let the pill packet rule your pill taking, not the bleeding pattern—whatever that may be. Do not stop taking pills before the end of a packet because of bleeding, even if it seems like a period. Pregnancies have happened that way.

Breakthrough bleeding (BTB)

> ## I am bleeding on days of pill taking: should I stop in the middle of a packet?
>
> The golden rule of pill taking is to carry on taking your pills according to the routine, irrespective of the pattern of bleeding or no-bleeding which may occur. Make an early appointment to discuss this with your doctor, particularly if it is a new problem or if you have been missing pills. They will look for other causes of bleeding, some of which have nothing to do with pill.

BTB starting in the first few months of use will almost always settle if you simply disregard it and continue to take the pills regularly, following the usual routine of 21 days on, 7 days off. Otherwise, after eliminating the obvious causes such as missed pills, vomiting, or the taking of an 'enzyme inducer' like St John's Wort—and whenever bleeding is a persistent or unexplained problem, or it occurs with intercourse—you should see your doctor soon. They may need to examine you and do some tests.

One quite common and potentially serious example that should be tested for is infection with chlamydia (see Glossary). Or there could be a polyp at the entrance to the uterus. Any treatment necessary would be simple and minor, often just as an out-patient. But if chlamydia is found, it is an STI so in addition any sexual contacts (either of you or of your partner) will need treatment too. If all other causes have been excluded (see Box 15.1), the dose of hormones may be too low. Try a phasic pill if you are on a monophasic; increase the progestogen

> ## Box 15.1 Causes of BTB on days of pill taking
>
> - *Disease*, e.g. chlamydia (see Glossary), can cause a blood-stained discharge.
> - *Disorders of pregnancy* that cause bleeding (e.g. recent miscarriage).
> - *Default*, i.e. missed pills; the resulting BTB may start 2 or 3 days afterwards, but can be very persistent thereafter.
> - *Drugs*, primarily enzyme inducers. Cigarettes can also cause BTB so stopping smoking can be one way of stopping the annoying symptom!
> - *Diarrhoea and/or vomiting*, diarrhoea alone has to be incredibly severe before it could make the pill fail.
> - *Duration of use too short*, i.e. within 2–3 months' use of any new pill brand.
> - *Dose*, after the above have been excluded.
>
> Modified from Sapire, E. (1990). *Contraception and Sexuality in Health and Disease*. New York: McGraw-Hill.

● **Bleeding on days of pill taking**
(i.e. breakthrough bleeding)

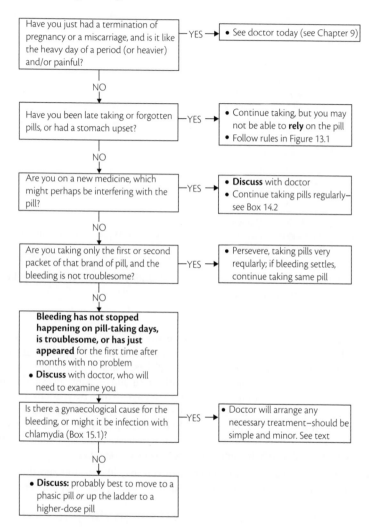

Figure 15.1a Which pill? Bleeding patterns (BTB).
Note: see Box 15.1—usefully referred to along with this figure.

● **No bleeding at all during pill-free
week** (no 'periods')—at least two missed*

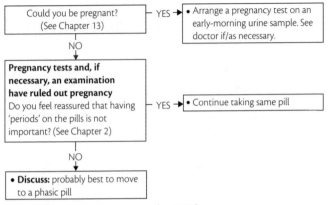

Figure 15.1b Which pill? Bleeding patterns (no WTB).
*Very important: if only one 'period' is missed and there is no reason to suspect failure of the pill, do not delay—start the next cycle of pills on the usual day.

component (or oestrogen if Loestrin 20®, Femodette®, or Mercilon® is being used); or try a different progestogen.

A missed 'period'

Consider Figure 15.1b. Have you forgotten any pills? Or has something else happened recently, like a bad stomach upset early in a packet, which might have reduced your protection against pregnancy? If there is any doubt, pregnancy must be ruled out by one or perhaps a series of urine tests and probably an examination. If you start getting symptoms such as nausea or pain, or miss two periods in a row, even if you are sure no pills were missed it is important to have a pregnancy test. If you do strongly suspect that you might be pregnant as a result of a pill-taking muddle, most doctors recommend that you transfer to using something like the condom method, carefully, until you know one way or another.

Once pregnancy has been ruled out, then you may like to stop and think if it really bothers you whether you get bleeding between packets of pills or not. If

> ### If I don't see much of a 'period' on the pill, or if I see no bleeding at all in the hormone-free week, is blood collecting inside me?
>
> No: if you have no bleeding it simply means that there is no blood to come away. After a check to make sure you are not pregnant, you can continue with the pill or other combined method if you wish.

you prefer to have your periods back, consider a phasic pill and then perhaps the brand on the next available rung up your particular ladder (see Chapter 16).

Nausea

Perseverance, or taking the pills with a drink and a little food at bedtime so that you are asleep when the symptom appears, is usually enough. Otherwise see your doctor or clinic, perhaps for a lower dose of oestrogen in the pill. Do not forget the possibility that the nausea might be due to pregnancy, of course, particularly if it appears for the first time after several months of not getting it. Arrange a pregnancy test if in any doubt.

Libido

Many women report that their sex lives improve once they go on the pill. Indeed most surveys have shown that pill users have more intercourse than non-users. This may be because the pill avoids the 'turn-off' effect which some couples find with alternative methods. Or it may reduce the regular loss of libido due to pre-menstrual symptoms that many women suffer in their 'normal' menstrual cycles.

But loss of libido is quite common and can be a real problem for some women. More often than not, it is has nothing to do with the pill. However, just as normal men have a little oestrogen in their blood, androgens are hormones produced in low amounts in women. Among other things, they help to promote normal sex drive. There are some pill brands (Dianette®, Yasmin®, and Yaz®) which contain progestogens that have *anti*-androgen effects. This makes them good for conditions such as acne, but if loss of libido came on after starting one of these it would be worth trying a brand containing a different progestogen.

I seem to have lost interest in sex. Should I stop the pill?

Only rarely should it be necessary for you to give up the pill solely because of loss of sex-drive. Could there be something wrong within your sexual relationship, for which some counselling might help? Could your loss of sex-drive be more to do with being depressed, in which case you should perhaps seek treatment primarily for that?

Vaginal discharge

A few women on the pill complain of excessive dryness of the vagina. This can be quite a problem for some, and may be partly responsible for a loss of interest in sex. It can be due to thrush (see below). Or it can mean that a pill with relatively too high a dose of progestogen is being used, in which case you could ask for a change of pill. It may also help to 'slow down', with a bit more foreplay before penetrative intercourse; or occasionally to use a lubricating jelly such as KY® or Sensilube®. Be straight with yourself, though, and with your partner. If the problem is more to do with some aspect of your sexual relationship, counselling would be more important than a change of pill brand or any lubricant.

Other women notice increased vaginal discharge. This is often due to *cervical ectopy*, or because of non-sexually transmitted vaginal infections such as *thrush* or *bacterial vaginosis*.

- Cervical ectopy is a harmless condition of the cervix, which is more common in pill users than in non-users. The outer surface of the cervix is normally covered by flattened cells, a little like normal skin. In contrast, the normal lining of the canal from the cervix into the main body of the uterus is upright, box-shaped cells with a lot of mucus-producing glands. If there is an ectopy, the normal glands lining the canal spread out over the outer part of the cervix. This means there are more mucus-producing glands and hence an increase in the normal wetness of the vagina. If the amount of discharge is a nuisance, perhaps requiring you to use a tampon or pad to control it, then your doctor can arrange very simple and painless out-patient treatment.

- Thrush—also known as candida or monilial infection—is due to a yeast, which usually lives in the vagina without causing any symptoms. Sometimes, it can cause an attack of intense itching of the vagina and vulva, with or very often without a curdy, white vaginal discharge. The pill does not cause thrush but it is more common in pregnancy, after antibiotics, and in women with diabetes. If you get thrush, on or off the pill, ask your pharmacist for some 'over-the-counter' treatment—usually pessaries and cream. There is also an oral treatment, useful particularly in resistant cases. In some women, thrush keeps recurring. They, and also their partners, may require extra help, perhaps from a GUM clinic.

- Bacterial vaginosis (BV) is due to bacteria that cause a fishy-smelling discharge and, like thrush, it has no known connection with the pill. The bacteria are treated with the antibiotic metronidazole.

Cystitis

If you get frequent bladder infections, see your doctor. There are some useful home treatments: for more on this ask for a leaflet about cystitis. It will probably help to empty your bladder both before and after intercourse and to use a lubricating jelly. You should take plenty of fluids—up to 3 litres in 3 hours—when you get an attack. Your doctor may sometimes advise taking a couple of antibiotic tablets shortly before intercourse as a regular preventive routine. Tests for vaginal infections such as thrush may also be necessary, as these infections can cause similar symptoms.

Other minor side-effects

These include breast tenderness or tingling, gain in weight, and leg aches and cramps. All these and more have been reported by pill users. However, every woman reacts in her own way, and the first pill tried is not always the best for you. As there are more than 20 varieties of combined pill, if you do have problems, it is usually possible to find a different brand that suits you better (see Chapter 16).

A very important point to remember is to give any particular brand a good try before giving up, and this usually means using it for at least 3 months. If either the bleeding or other types of minor side-effects occur, they usually do settle down after the first two or three courses of pills.

Serious side-effects: reasons to stop the pill at once

Box 15.2 lists symptoms which, though most unlikely to occur, should lead you to contact a doctor at once and to inform him or her that you are taking the pill.

Box 15.2 Important symptoms and situations meaning 'stop the pill'

- Severe pain in the calf of one leg, especially if linked with swelling (not the aching legs that so many people get, nor simple painless swelling of *both* ankles).
- Severe central pain in the chest, or severe sharp pains in either side of the chest, aggravated by breathing.
- Unexplained breathlessness, or cough with blood-stained phlegm.
- Severe pain in the abdomen.
- Any unusually severe, prolonged headache, particularly migraine, especially if it is the first-ever such attack, or is very different from previous ones, or gets worse with the passage of time, or keeps returning.
- Loss of part of the field of vision, right or left, either blackness or not; and if not black maybe with a bright zigzag line round it, usually but not necessarily *followed by* a one-sided headache (migraine with aura).
- *Marked* numbness and tingling coming on quickly to affect one side of the body (e.g. one arm, or the side of the tongue).
- Sudden disturbance of the ability to speak normally.
- A bad fainting attack, or vertigo, or first-ever epileptic fit.
- A severe and generalized, perhaps painful, skin rash.
- Jaundice—yellow eyes and skin.
- If found to have a very high blood pressure.
- Admission as an emergency to a hospital bed after an accident, or for a major operation (see Chapter 9).
- Any other kind of immobilization, for any reason—especially for a broken bone or badly torn ligaments in your leg.

They may or may not mean anything serious or even be anything to do with the pill but it is best to play safe. They are the only reasons for stopping immediately, wherever you are in a pack.

What to do?

The symptoms in Box 15.2 mean that any pill user should:

- Stop the pill until further notice, transferring to another effective method of contraception.
- Seek medical advice without delay, so that the right diagnosis can be made and any necessary treatment started.

Importantly, the vast majority of pill takers go for years and years without getting a single frightening symptom. And even the ones above may well have a cause that is nothing to do with the pill. If the doctor is able to reassure you that a symptom from the list above is not relevant to pill taking, you can restart following the rules for missed pills (Chapter 13).

I am going skiing and I take the pill. What should I do if I break a leg?

Most people realize that the pill should be stopped if you become suddenly bed-bound due to illness, accident, or major surgery as an emergency. But not enough know that even if a leg only has to be pinned or completely fixed in plaster after a fracture, once again the pill—or EVRA®, or NuvaRing®—should be avoided or stopped. There is a real risk of thrombosis in that leg: so as well as stopping the combined hormonal method immediately, inform the surgeon who will probably decide to give you blood-thinning (anti-coagulant) medication—if s/he wasn't going to anyway.

16

Which pill should I choose?

Key points

◆ Almost all pills contain ethinylestradiol (EE), a synthetic oestrogen, in differing doses.

◆ Different progestogens can affect the 'potency' of oestrogen.

◆ Certain combinations of oestrogen and progestogen may suit different women with specific conditions.

Table 16.1 lists the many varieties of pills that are currently available in the UK. You can visit http://www.ippf.org.uk for the formulations and equivalent names of all the hormonal contraceptives that are in use anywhere, in all other countries of the world. One main oestrogen, EE, is used everywhere, but there are several different progestogens.

Pill ladders

Figure 16.1. shows the different progestogens in each of the fixed-dose combined and progestogen-only pills available in the UK. Those providing the same progestogen in each of the groups A–F have been arranged in ladders.

The effects of different progestogens on blood clotting were discussed in Chapter 7. Essentially, there are two main groups of progestogens, shown in Figure 16.1:

◆ Less 'oestrogen-dominant': a smaller group with two progestogens, LNG and NET, that seem to oppose the oestrogen effects but consequently are more likely to have side-effects of greasiness of hair and skin, and acne (or at least fail to improve these symptoms as much as oestrogen-dominant pills do).

◆ More 'oestrogen-dominant': containing the progestogens DSG, GSD, NGM, and DSP. These pills are sometimes chosen from the start for some reason, e.g. if acne is a big problem, but they are more normally tried second, when the first choice has not suited.

Table 16.1 Combined pills with less than 50 mcg of oestrogen available in the UK

Name of pill	Dose of oestrogen (EE) (mcg)	Name and dose of progestogen (mcg)	Remarks
Group A		**Drospirenone (DSP)**	
Yasmin°	30	3000	
Yaz°	20	3000	24/4 system
Group B		**Norgestimate (NGM)**	**EVRA° is similar**
Cilest°	35	250	
Group C		**Gestodene (GSD)**	
Femodene°/ Femodene ED° Katya°	30	75	
Femodette° Sunya 20/75°	20	75	
Triadene°	30, 40, 30 [32.4]	50, 70, 100 [79]	Triphasic: doses are for 6, 5, then 10 days, respectively
Group D		**Desogestrel (DSG)**	
Marvelon°	30	150	
Mercilon°	20	150	Nuva Ring° is similar
Group E		**Levonorgestrel (LNG)**	
Ovranette° Microgynon 30°/ Microgynon 30 ED°	30	150	
Logynon°/ Logynon ED°	30, 40, 30 [32.4]	50, 75, 125 [92]	Triphasic: doses are for 6, 5, then 10 days, respectively
Group F		**Norethisterone (NET)**	
Binovum°	35, 35, [35]	500, 1000 [833]	Biphasic: doses are for 7 then 14 days, respectively
Loestrin 30°	30	1500	
Loestrin 20°	20	1000	
Norimin°	35	1000	
Brevinor° Ovysmen°	35	500	

Table 16.1 Combined pills with less than 50 mcg of oestrogen available in the UK *(continued)*

Name of pill	Dose of oestrogen (EE) (mcg)	Name and dose of progestogen (mcg)	Remarks
Synphase®	35, 35, 35 [35]	500, 1000, 500 [714]	Triphasic: doses are for 7, 9, then 5 days
Trinovum®	35, 35, 35 [35]	500, 750, 1000 [750]	Triphasic: each dose for 7 days

Notes:

1. Each group uses a different progestogen. All are 21/7 systems unless stated otherwise.

2. The pills bracketed together have identical formulas, but are marketed by different companies.

3. Average daily doses of phasic pills are in square brackets.

4. ED versions have seven blank or dummy tablets of lactose for the no-treatment days.

5. Although Yaz® is fully approved, UK marketing has been delayed (see Foreword).

6. Qlaira® is a new (2009) and very different phasic product: it uses *natural* oestrogen combined with a progestogen that is new to the UK (see p.133). It contains oestradiol valerate (E2V) with dienogest (DNG) in 4 phases over 26 days, plus just 2 dummy reminder tablets. Phase 1: 2 tablets E2V 3000 mcg (dark yellow); phase 2: 5 tablets E2V 2000 mcg + DNG 2000 mcg (medium red); phase 3: 17 tablets E2V 2000 mcg + DNG 3000 mcg (light yellow); phase 4: 2 tablets E2V 1000 mcg (dark red); finally: 2 tablets Lactose (white).

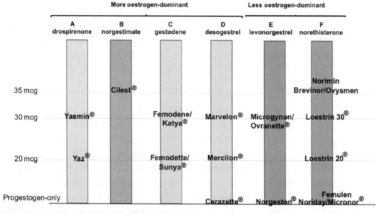

Figure 16.1 Pill ladders (excluding phasic pills).

What about Yasmin® and Yaz®?

Both pills contain DSP together with EE. Yasmin® contains 30 mcg of EE taken 21/7, while Yaz® contains 20 mcg of EE taken for 24 days followed by only a 4-day break (24/4). DSP differs from other progestogens in pills because:

◆ It is an anti-androgen, and the combination is also oestrogen-dominant, making it a good alternative to the well-known Dianette® for the treatment of moderately bad acne and the PCOS.

◆ It is a weak diuretic, meaning it makes the kidney get rid of more fluid from the body. This makes it a useful second choice to try for some minor side-effects, particularly for women who have premenstrual symptoms of fluid retention such as bloatedness and cyclical breast enlargement.

What about Dianette® (co-cyprindiol)?

There is a fifth progestogen (cyproterone acetate, an anti-androgen) in the 'oestrogen-dominant' group, which is not among the ladders in Figure 16.1— only because it is on the market as a treatment, not as a 'routine' pill.

Dianette® or co-cyprindiol (cyproterone acetate 2 mg with EE 35 mcg) is licensed for the treatment of severe acne and moderately severe hirsutism. But practically everything else, good and bad, about ordinary (oestrogen-dominant) pills in this book applies also to Dianette®.

Can I take Dianette® long-term for my skin?

For women with known hyperandrogenism who attend specialist clinics, Dianette® may be the only effective treatment for severe symptoms. Most women will be able to stop Dianette® 3–4 months after resolution of symptoms (not 3–4 months of treatment). In practice, many women find that Yasmin® or Yaz® are well able to control milder acne either from the beginning or once it has first been controlled by Dianette®. If these alternatives are not effective, Dianette® can be re-prescribed in the longer-term with regular review.

Phasic pills: triphasic or biphasic brands

Everything written so far also applies to phasic pills, since the actual hormones they contain are not different. All are low-dose varieties in which the ratio of the progestogen to the oestrogen is not fixed, as normally, but is made to change at least once during each 21-day course of pills. There is a stepwise increase in the progestogen dose at each change, so that there is less in the first phase than in the second (biphasic pills), or in the second and usually the third phases (triphasic pills). There are six brands in all (details in Table 16.1), one of which (BiNovum®) is biphasic and five are triphasic. The advantages and disadvantages are listed in Box 16.1; they are mainly used as second-choice pills if fixed-dose pills are not satisfactory.

Tailoring the pill to you

All marketed pills are options from the start. LNG pills such as Microgynon® are usually prescribed for first-time users, since they suit most people, most of the time. But it is impossible to predict which pill will suit which woman, so whichever pill you start with, it's your choice to switch. As always, 'the informed user should be the chooser'.

Box 16.1 Advantages and disadvantage of phasic pills

Advantages

- They are almost 100 per cent effective, like other pills, if taken regularly.
- There is usually good control of the bleeding pattern—especially in some women who have great difficulty with all other products.
- They are particularly 'good' at giving a definite 'withdrawal bleed'.

Disadvantages

- There is a reduced margin for error if women forget pills in the first week of a pack, after the 'contraception-free' time.
- There is some evidence that pill-taking errors are actually more common, as some versions do not have the day of the week against the tablet and there are two or three phases (or even four in ED versions) to take in the right order.
- Explaining how to use them takes a bit more of the doctor's or nurse's time.
- Some women complain of premenstrual symptoms, such as breast tenderness, during the final phase of pill taking.
- Headaches and other symptoms brought on by hormone fluctuations are possible.
- Bleeding can be heavier and more painful than fixed-dose pills.
- They are not suitable for tricycling.

Women vary considerably, in the way their bodies absorb and react to the pill's hormones, and very different blood hormone levels have been found. A likely conclusion is that many unwanted effects, both serious and 'minor', are connected with having unnecessarily high blood hormone levels—caused either by unusually efficient absorption or inefficient elimination of the hormones. On the other hand, the problem of BTB or spotting can be linked with quite the opposite: too low blood levels reaching the womb's lining.

Since it is impractical to measure blood hormone levels routinely, doctors have tended in the past to give some women more hormone than might have been necessary. To make this less likely, new prescriptions should generally start with a brand of pills from near the bottom of one of the ladders. This policy will still provide women with adequate protection against pregnancy, but might result in problems with their bleeding pattern. These can be managed, along with other side-effects, by forewarning, and by following the advice in Chapter 13.

If the first pill does not suit, which should be the second choice?

Problems with the bleeding cycle

All other causes of BTB in Chapter 15 must first have been ruled out. The problem can then often be solved by a change of pill. You might shift to using one of the phasic pills; or otherwise try moving 'up the ladder' to another pill containing the same hormones as the one which you are presumably finding satisfactory except for this bleeding problem. For example, if you were to develop BTB or spotting with Ovysmen®/Brevinor® in ladder F, your doctor might suggest Norimin®. A pill taker with a bit of acne who was taking Mercilon® could go on to Marvelon®, or try Cilest®, Femodene®/Katya®, or Yaz® from different ladders.

Similarly, if you are bothered by absent withdrawal bleeds on your present pill, consider a phasic pill and then perhaps the brand on the next available rung up your particular ladder.

Other side-effects

If you have a symptom that could perhaps be serious (see the list in Chapter 13), or if you are not quite sure that it is not one of those, you should contact your doctor today and take no further pills unless the doctor says that you may. Otherwise, follow the advice in Fig. 16.2.

There are many other less serious but annoying non-bleeding side-effects that pill takers may get: nausea, weight gain, breast symptoms, headaches which are not 'migraine with aura', mood changes and depression, acne—and there are others discussed in Chapter 6. If such side-effects continue beyond the two or three courses of pills which are often necessary to give your body a chance to get used to any particular brand, or much sooner if you find the symptom cannot be tolerated, then there are two possibilities (Box 16.2).

Box 16.2 Managing side-effects

First, you could ask to move further down your current ladder, provided there is a pill brand available that contains even less hormone (remember to skip the pill break when you start the lower dose pill).

Secondly, if:

- there is no room for you to go down more rungs on a particular ladder, or
- doing that causes BTB, or
- it seems possible that your side-effect is due to a particular progestogen

then consider a 'sideways shift'. This means moving to a different ladder altogether and starting to take a pill that contains a different progestogen.

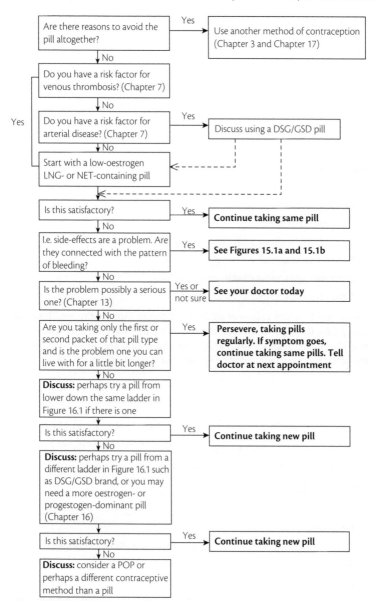

Figure 16.2 Which pill?

Note: 'Discuss' means discuss at next visit with doctor or nurse: they will not take kindly to being told by you what to do next. If moving down a ladder, start the new packet without any break (see Chapter 15).

See Boxes 16.3 and 16.4 for some more specific (though not fully scientifically proven) guidelines. These may sometimes be helpful in deciding which pill to try next.

Box 16.3 Conditions linked with relative progestogen excess may be helped by a more oestrogen-dominant pill (pills not containing LNG or NET)

Some cases of:

- Dryness of vagina.
- Sustained weight gain.
- Depression/tiredness.
- Loss of libido along with depressed mood.
- Breast tenderness.
- Acne and greasiness of skin and head hair.
- Unwanted hair growth (hirsutism).

There may be other causes of all these problems. Among the low-dose combined pills the most oestrogen-dominant formulae seem to be Marvelon® and Cilest®. Yasmin® (or Yaz®) and Dianette® are often successful in moderately severe cases of acne or hirsutism, especially in PCOS.

Box 16.4 Some conditions linked with relative oestrogen excess may be helped by a more progestogen-dominant pill (containing LNG or NET)

- Nausea.
- Dizziness.
- Feelings of bloating/cyclical weight gain due to fluid retention.
- Vaginal discharge (no infection present).
- Some cases of breast pain with enlargement.
- Some cases of lost libido without depression, especially if taking an anti-androgen (Yasmin®, Yaz®, or Dianette®).
- Growth of breast lumps.

- Growth of fibroids.
- Endometriosis.

As before, there may be other causes, but for any of the above problems it is often worth trying a pill with the lowest possible dose of oestrogen combined with relatively more progestogen. Lowering the oestrogen (e.g. Marvelon® to Mercilon®) is one possibility, otherwise Microgynon 30®/Ovranette® would be appropriate.

Since starting on the pill, I feel sick and dizzy and have too much vaginal discharge—what shall I do?

All these may well improve after two or three courses of pills. Nausea is often worse in the first few days after each pill-free interval, but then happens on fewer and fewer days with each new packet. It can also often be reduced by taking the pills last thing at night.

Otherwise these and related symptoms, which seem to be due to too much oestrogen effect in comparison with the progestogen effect, can be helped by using a progestogen-dominant pill (Box 16.4), or by the progestogen-only pill (e.g. Cerazette®).

New combined pill-type methods: including new routes of delivery for hormones

Qlaira®: innovative new phasic pill with natural oestrogen

Though still a pill, this is new (2009) and different. Its progestogen called dienogest (DNG) is new to the UK, though it has been used successfully for many years in Eastern Europe in a monophasic combined pill called Valette®. It also is the first contraceptive to use oestradiol valerate (E2V) which, after it is swallowed, is rapidly converted into oestradiol – the main 'natural' oestrogen produced by the ovaries in a normal menstrual cycle (Chapter 2). Because of this, in order to give the user of Qlaira a good bleeding cycle it has to be given in a uniquely different way, in four different phases during 26 days followed by just 2 dummy tablets (Table 16.1), with a new pack then started immediately, without a break. The advice to follow if pills are missed is therefore also a bit different (read the leaflet supplied with each packet). The combination has less effect on some of the important substances made in the liver (Table 4.1) including some of the clotting factors, so it is hoped but not yet proven that this will make it even less likely than other pills to cause circulatory problems (Chapter 7). But Qlaira is so new that it will take a while for us to know all its pros and cons – watch this space!

EVRA® skin patch: the transdermal route

This is an innovative skin patch delivering EE with norelgestromin, the name for the active progestogen hormone produced in the body out of the NGM contained in a tablet of Cilest®. Indeed, in an oversimplified way, you can say that using EVRA® is a bit like taking 'Cilest® through the skin'.

Each patch is worn for 7 days for three consecutive weeks followed by a patch-free week, during which the bleed happens (often starting later than with the pill and lasting till after the day you must put on the next patch). If wanted, bleeds can be easily postponed by just skipping a patch-free week, just as with pills.

Like any version of the combined pill containing oestrogen, it might still cause rare serious side-effects such as thrombosis. All the advice in earlier chapters about the pill also applies to EVRA®, with some obvious minor differences. It seems to be relatively oestrogen-dominant, and has bleeding and non-bleeding side-effects very like Cilest® itself. About 2 per cent of women in the trials had local skin reactions bad enough to make them give it up. Otherwise, the patch sticks really well, even in hot climates and in the gym or when bathing or showering. In the trials, overall 1.8 per cent of patches fell off and 2.9 per cent became partially detached. Its effectiveness (see Box 16.5) is similar to the oral pills overall—the failure rate being less than one per 100 woman-years.

Box 16.5 Ensuring EVRA® is effective

- Avoid use at all if your body weight is greater than 90 kg, since it has a higher failure rate. It is not a good choice anyway if there is any risk factor for VTE.

- Be aware that the contraceptive is in the glue of the patch, so a dry patch that has fallen off should not be reused!

- As with the ordinary pill it is *essential* never to lengthen the contraception-free time, which is the patch-free time. If this interval exceeds 8 days for any reason (either through late application or the first new patch detaching and this being identified late) use extra precautions for the duration of the first newly applied patch (i.e. for 7 days) and, if you had sex in the patch-free days, best take immediate emergency contraception as well.

- Absorption problems through vomiting/diarrhoea, and taking the antibiotic tetracycline by mouth, do not affect this method's effectiveness.

- During any short-term enzyme inducer treatment, and as usual for 28 days after this ends, additional contraception is advised plus elimination of any patch-free intervals during this time. EVRA® is only recommended for long-term use during such treatment if the user is prepared to continue always using condoms as well.

EVRA® needs to be disposed of properly to avoid potential water pollution by its hormones, i.e. not down the toilet, sealing it with the sticky label provided.

If it's so like the pill, why bother using the patch? The patch is most useful for women who find it difficult to remember a daily pill, especially as if the patch-user does forget, there is a 2-day margin for error for late patch change (i.e. it still works up to 9 days).

NuvaRing®: transvaginal combined hormonal contraception

This combined vaginal ring releases etonogestrel, which is the active substance in the body after swallowing DSG. It gives a dose of 120 mcg along with EE 15 mcg per day, so thus ends up very like 'vaginal Mercilon®'. It is normally retained for 3 weeks and then taken out for the withdrawal bleeding during the fourth week. At the woman's choice this bleed could be missed by putting in her next month's ring straightaway, with no break. Like Evra®, an advantage is that it may help women with a bad memory for taking pills.

Most men don't notice NuvaRing® during sex, but it can be removed, rinsed in warm water, and reinserted up to 3 hours later without having to use extra precautions. Expulsion is an additional problem potentially affecting efficacy (see Box 16.6).

For the time being we must assume that it has about the same risk as Mercilon® of serious side-effects such as thrombosis. Moreover, all advice about the pill earlier in this book must be presumed to apply to NuvaRing®. It appears to have a minor side-effect rate very like that of Mercilon itself.

Box 16.6 Ensuring NuvaRing® is effective

♦ Expulsion is a problem for some women, especially those who have had babies. This happens mainly during the emptying of bowels or bladder, so the women therefore easily notices this and could take steps to avoid the method failing. Since it is so unobtrusive and could get forgotton, you should check regularly that it's there – especially after the ring-free time.

♦ As with the COC, it is still absolutely essential never to lengthen the contraception-free (ring-free) interval. If this interval exceeds 8 days for any reason use extra precautions for the first 7 days and, if you had sex during the ring-free interval, take immediate emergency contraception.

♦ Absorption problems, vomiting/diarrhoea, and broad-spectrum anti-biotics such as tetracycline have no effect on this method's efficacy.

♦ If there needs to be enzyme inducer treatment, we would advise additional contraception and missing the ring-free intervals—but an IUD, IUS, or the injection would be even better.

Part 4

Other types of pill

17

The progestogen-only pill

> **→ Key points**
>
> ◆ The POP contains only one hormone—progestogen.
>
> ◆ The POP is very suited to women who prefer to take pills but cannot, or do not wish to take, oestrogen.
>
> ◆ There are two main types, the standard POP (mini-pill) and Cerazette®, which prevent pregnancy in different ways.
>
> ◆ The failure rate ranges from <1–1 per 100 women per year for Cerazette® and from 1–4 per 100 woman-years for the standard POP.
>
> ◆ Side-effects are few and mostly relate to a disrupted bleeding pattern.

POPs, previously known as 'mini-pills' are *not* versions of the COC. They do not contain any oestrogen and the progestogen itself is generally also in a lower dose than in combined pills. Unlike combined pills, POPs are taken every day, including during periods. POPs have very little effect on your body chemistry, so can be taken safely by many women who are unable to take COCs. Just as with COCs, an overdose of POPs can cause no serious harm to an adult or child. Types of POP available in the UK are shown in Table 17.1. If you live in another country, you can refer to http://www.ippf.org.uk to compare the locay avaiabe brands of POP.

The POP can be particularly valuable for:

◆ Women who are breastfeeding.

◆ Women with risk factors for using, or side-effects on, the COC. Weight gain, nausea, mood problems and depression, and headaches all seem to be helped by this move.

◆ Women who have migraine with aura.

◆ Blood pressure problems on the COC pill.

◆ Diabetics.

Table 17.1 POPs available in the UK

Name of pill	No. in packet	Name and dose of progestogen (mcg)	Remarks
Group D		Desogestrel	
Cerazette®	28	75	Blocks egg release more often than the other POPs
Group E		Levonorgestrel	
Norgeston®	35	30	
Group F		Norethisterone	
Micronor® Noriday®	28	350	
Femulen®	28	500	Contains etynodiol diacetate which converts to norethisterone in the body

Note: groups contain the same progestogens as the groups with the same letter in Table 16.1 and Figure 16.1.

- Obesity, with a BMI over 30 and especially 40 and above (best choice being Cerazette®).
- Smokers, especially over age 35.
- Other older women, especially non-smokers around the menopause.

Who should avoid the POP?

Conditions in which to avoid standard POPs and Cerazette®

- Any serious side-effect on the combined pill which was not clearly due to oestrogen—e.g. past liver tumour, allergy to progestogen itself.
- Breast cancer if recent—see below.
- Undiagnosed bleeding.
- Actual or possible pregnancy.
- Any condition that significantly interferes with the POP being absorbed—e.g. Crohn's disease.

Conditions in which standard POPs and Cerazette® can be used with caution

- Breast cancer—if in remission, with no probems for years (typically 5 years) past, in consultation with the cancer speciaist.
- High risk or past history of thrombosis in an artery—due to concern about sight unwanted effects on bood fats.
- Enzyme-inducing medicine—Cerazette® and we would advise two tablets a day on a 'named patient' basis.
- Cysts on the ovary—if history of pain.
- Past ectopic pregnancy—standard POP only but no restriction for Cerazette®.

- Past venous thrombosis or risk factors for VTE.
- Risk factors for arteria disease.
- Amost a ong-term diseases—incuding iver damage with abnorma bood test eves.

How do POPs work?

Standard POPs do not rely entirely on stopping release of the egg. As a result, most periods that a woman gets on this pill, unlike those on COCs, are natural ones. The POP's main effect is to interfere with the passage of sperm through the mucus at the entrance to the uterus (cervix). The slippery mucus normally released under the influence of oestrogen is altered by the artificial progesterone and becomes a scanty and thick material, creating an effective barrier to the sperm. This happens whether or not the POP prevents egg release that month which it does about half the time—more in long-term or older users.

Even the small amount of hormone present in the POP can be enough to stop egg release, and this is even more likely with Cerazette®. It means two things: the hypothalamus and pituitary in the brain are being made inactive by this

Table 17.2 How POPs prevent pregnancy

	Combined pills	Standard POPs	Cerazette®
1. Reduced FSH therefore follicles stopped from ripening and egg from maturing	+ + + +	+ +	+ + + +
2. LH surge stopped so no egg release	+ + + +	+ +	+ + + +
3. Cervical mucus changed into a barrier to sperm	+ + +	+ + +	+ + +
4. Lining of uterus made less suitable for implantation of an embryo (uncertainty whether this effect is sufficient alone to stop a conception)	+	+	+
5. Uterine tubes perhaps affected so that they do not transport egg so well (uncertainty about this also)	+	+	+
Expected pregnancy rate per 100 women using the pill method consistently for 1 year (compare use of 'No method' = 80–90)	<1	1–4	<1

Notes:

1. The more plus signs the greater the effect.

2. The standard POP disturbs or prevents egg release (effect 2) in over half of all POP users increasingly with increased duration of use. Women with regular cycles are more likely to be relying on effect 3.

3. If taken when breastfeeding, standard POPs have a similar mode of action to Cerazette®.

low dose of a single hormone in the same way as happens in any woman who is taking any combined pill. *No egg release means you are as protected against pregnancy as if you were on the combined pill* (without taking the known [small] risks of oestrogen)!

When to choose Cerazette®

There are situations in which women need the efficacy of the combined pill but without the oestrogen. These include:

◆ Young, fertile women—especially if they are at all forgetful.

◆ Young woman with complicated structural heart disease—who should avoid oestrogen; in such cases a pregnancy might be unusually risky.

◆ COC users waiting for major or leg surgery.

◆ Women who might especially benefit from a method which blocks ovulation (egg release)—e.g. past history of an ectopic pregnancy or menstrual problems that are more usually treated by the COC, such as painful or heavy periods, PMS, or breast tenderness.

◆ Women who weigh more than 70 kg—given also that any POP is safer than a COC for women with a high BMI.

Side-effects of the POP

Though little research has been done, what we do know about unwanted side-effects is reassuring when compared with our knowledge about the combined pill. Any important increase in *cancer risk* is believed unlikely (though not *proven*). If you develop a problem with the cycle or any other side-effect with one POP, and still wish to use the method, then it is certainly worth switching to one of the others.

Bleeding

An erratic bleeding pattern is the biggest problem, particularly with Cerazette®. Although some of the bleeds that happen are periods caused the normal way, the progestogen can, and often does, affect the bleeding mechanisms of the lining of the uterus. So, women can have more frequent bleeds; longer or shorter than before; very irregular; or relatively regular with frequent and unexpected extra bleeds from the lining of the uterus in between the periods. If you persevere, the menstrual pattern normally becomes acceptable after a few months. In the studies of Cerazette® there was a trend for the more annoying frequent and prolonged bleeding to lessen with time: at 1 year around 50 per cent of the women had either only one or two bleeds per 90 days.

Premenstrual symptoms

Premenstrual symptoms are very variable, depending on how much the cycle is altered by the POP. Symptoms are usually unchanged, but in different women they can be either worsened or improved.

Other effects

A much smaller proportion of women than is found on the combined pill complain of things such as *weight gain*, *loss of libido*, *headaches*, and *dizziness*. As with the combined pill, these symptoms are usually only a problem in the first 2 or 3 months, and it is worth persevering at least that long, as they could well disappear. A few women also complain of *acne*. Pain caused by *cysts on the ovary* can occur with all POPs, including Cerazette®, though more often such cysts give no symptoms. Unlike the combined pill, POPs make cysts more likely to be formed.

Ectopic pregnancy

Ectopics are rare, but serious, as the pregnancy cannot continue normally and may eventually break into a blood vessel. It starts with severe pain in the lower abdomen, usually on one side or the other, not coming and going like normal menstrual cramps. If the cause is an ectopic, the period will generally be a few days overdue, or you may have had what seemed like a prolonged and lighter-than-usual period. However, even without that history, when in doubt you should see *and be examined by* a doctor. If you have a positive urine pregnancy test and they feel it possible that the pregnancy is in the tube—it can often be very difficult to be sure—then you will be referred to the nearest hospital for further tests and possibly an operation if required.

Even in POP users the actual cause of virtually all ectopic pregnancies is not the POP: it is damage to a tube by an earlier pelvic infection, most commonly with chlamydia (see Glossary). Since on the standard POP (unlike the combined pill) egg release can still occur, a sperm may manage to get through the barrier of altered cervical mucus and fertilize an egg; and then, because of the damaged tube, the early embryo may get stuck and grow there rather than on the wall of the uterus. Because of this, although ectopics are overall *less* likely in POP users than among women not using contraception, among the very few failures that happen the standard POP is less good at stopping an ectopic pregnancy from resulting.

This is not a problem with Cerazette®: because of its very strong ability to stop egg release, it is equally good at stopping ectopics and womb pregnancies. So it is a better choice than a standard POP to reduce the risk of another ectopic in someone who already had one in the past.

Taking POPs

POPs need to be taken meticulously, though Cerazette® is more forgiving. It is very important to take your standard POP at the same hour of each day. The mucus effect seems to be lost if you are just 3 hours late, i.e. just 27 hours since the last tablet. It's not easy to be so meticulous, so set a dedicated alarm on your mobile!

> **Myth:** You need to take the POP around 4 hours before you usually have sex.
>
> **Fact:** Pill taking can be at any time of day, a time of your own choosing.

You take your first tablet of any POP on the first day of a period, and start each subsequent packet immediately following the last tablet of the one before. With a day 1 start, no extra contraceptive precautions need be taken.

Miscarriage or termination of pregnancy

Start immediately; no extra precautions are required.

After delivery of a baby

POPs do not increase the risk of blood clots (thrombosis). So they *can* be started straight away. However, extra bleeding or spotting can be caused by an early start even if you breastfeed and expect no periods: so it is usually better to start on about day 21 after the delivery. No extra precautions are required, even if you do not breastfeed.

If you start later, before periods have returned, you need first to rule out another pregnancy by a urine test. You can then start the POP but allow 7 days for the full build-up of the contraception before having unprotected sex.

From the COC to the POP

Take the first pill from the POP packet the day after the last combined pill. As there is some 'carry-over' of the latter's contraceptive effects, it is then unnecessary to use another method initially as well.

From the POP to the COC, or another family-planning method

It is best to have the first packet of the combined pill ready, and to transfer directly to it, on the first day of your next definite period, perhaps before you have finished the final POP packet. This is also the best time to stop if you are transferring to a method such as the condom or the cap. The reason is that waiting to the end of your POP packet might coincide with egg release, at the most fertile time 2 weeks before the next period—not a good time for changing methods.

If you do not see any periods at all, then you could wait until the end of your current packet before taking the first COC, or starting another new method. Either way you can assume continuous protection against pregnancy.

Missed POPs

There is a lot less 'margin' with standard POPs than with Carazette® (see Boxes 17.1 and 17.2). In all of the following circumstances—missing pills, stomach upsets (vomiting), the use of interfering drugs—loss of protection against pregnancy is more likely and more immediate than with the combined pill. You are also more likely to get irregular bleeding, which is in any case a more common problem on any POP. Fortunately it takes just two days for the mucus barrier to get fully restored by the POP.

Box 17.1 The standard POP and missed pills

If you are more than 3 hours late in taking the standard POP:

- Take the one(s) you have missed **and**
- Abstain or use condoms for two complete days (48 hours), during which you have taken two daily tablets correctly.

If you vomit a newly taken pill within 2 hours:

- Replace the vomited pill (or pills, if it was a long vomiting attack) with tablets from the end of your current pack, or a spare one, so you can keep the days of the week of your pill taking right.

- Abstain or use another method like the condom for two complete days (48 hours), during which you have taken two daily tablets correctly.

If you've already had sex with no condom during this time (including the 48 hours after restarting tablet taking), you may also need emergency contraception (see Chapter 19).

Box 17.2 Cerazette® and missed pills

If you are more than 12 hours late in taking Cerazette®:

- Take the one(s) you have missed **and**
- Abstain or use another method for two complete days (48 hours), during which you have taken two daily tablets correctly.

If you vomit a newly taken pill within two hours:

- Replace the vomited pill (or pills, if it was a long vomiting attack) with tablets from the end of your current pack, or a spare one, so you can keep the days of the week of your pill taking right.

- If the replacement pill was more than 12 hours from the usual time for pill taking, abstain or use another method for two complete days (48 hours), during which you have taken two daily tablets correctly.

If you've already had sex with no condom during this time (including the 48 hours after restarting tablet taking), you may also need emergency contraception (see Chapter 19).

Cerazette® primarily blocks egg release and relies very rarely on the sperm-blocking mucus effect. This means that you have much more leeway (12 hours instead of 3) but otherwise the same rules apply as for standard POPs.

What about interactions between POPs and other medicines?

Ordinary antibiotics are not a problem with this pill. This is because progestogen blood levels are not dependent on the recycling process from the large bowel, which happens only with oestrogens. But the medicines called enzyme inducers that can make the liver eliminate both the COC's hormones faster from the blood also reduce the effectiveness of the one hormone in POPs. So extra precautions *do* need to be used during short courses of such treatment (and for up to 4 weeks thereafter since their effects are long-lasting).

Women with epilepsy or others who have to be on an enzyme-inducing drug long-term should preferably use another method, such as an injectable, IUD, or IUS. But if nothing else suits, your doctor may suggest two Cerazette® tablets a day (on the so-called 'named patient' basis) to restore effectiveness.

How reversible is the POP?

As the dose of hormone is so low, return of fertility with all POPs, including Cerazette®, is rapid. Indeed, if continuing to avoid a conception is vital for you, becoming fertile again must be assumed to be almost immediate.

After stopping this pill, your fertility should be just the same as it would have been at your (now a bit older) age if you had never taken it. Remember though, that at least one in eight of all couples experience delay or may need some treatment before they achieve a pregnancy.

If while taking the POP you go on seeing periods, this is almost a test of fertility, as it probably means that, in spite of taking the artificial hormone, you are able to continue to have egg release and natural periods.

How do you know when you have reached the menopause?

If the older POP user has no periods, it can be quite difficult to know if the menopause has actually happened, though a blood test can sometimes help. A low value of the hormone FSH from the pituitary gland suggests that the lack of periods is just because of the POP and that you still need to take it. High values of FSH are suggestive of being at or around the menopause, especially if you have hot flushes as well. Unfortunately, the only proof that you can no longer conceive is after a whole year without periods when no hormones are being taken. This is because late ovulations can still occur, even when the periods seem to have stopped.

> Margaret's periods stopped when she was 50. She was taking the standard POP and the doctor suggested that she could stop it and just use spermicide for 1 year, provided that she had no further bleeding. Margaret wasn't keen on spermicides, which she perceived as being messy, and felt that the POP suited her well. Her doctor suggested that she could continue the standard POP until she was 56, which is 5 years after the average age of the final period. By that time, she could be sure that her ovaries had completely stopped working.

What about overweight women?

Some research suggested that the standard POP may be more likely to fail in women over 70 kg (11 stone), regardless of their height, so the UK FPA has for some years warned of a possibly increased failure rate. Cerazette® would be a good first choice of POP for this group of women, because anovulant hormonal methods (those that primarily stop egg release) have generally been found not to lose their effectiveness to any important extent as weight goes up, at least to 90 kg.

What about breastfeeding?

Unlike COCs, POPs do not interfere at all with the quantity or significantly with the quality of breast milk. Breastfeeding under certain conditions has a good contraceptive effect on its own. So in combination with the standard POP the efficacy is likely to be the same as if you were not breastfeeding and took Cerazette®. If a mother who breastfeeds chooses the standard POP, in the UK she is usually advised to start on about the 21st day following delivery. However, since risk of conception early on in full breastfeeding is so low, you can wait to start the POP when the baby is 6 weeks old.

How much of the POP does the baby get?

A very tiny amount of the hormone in all POPs has been shown to get into the milk, the least being found in milk from women who use pills containing only levonorgestrel—meaning Norgeston®. This transfer via milk to infant causes concern to some mothers, but there is absolutely no evidence that this amount of hormone has ever harmed any baby. After more than 2 years of full breastfeeding, the infant of a mother using these POPs will have taken the equivalent of just one tablet.

What about weaning?

When you decide to cut down on the breastfeeding, and especially when your first period comes on, you may like to change to Cerazette®, or to a low-dose combined pill, or perhaps use an injectable or implant. This is important for extra reliability when you lose the contraceptive effect of breastfeeding. Or you could choose a non-hormonal method right through, such as an IUD or condoms. *It's your call*—as contraception always should be!

18

Emergency contraception

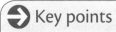 Key points

- Emergency hormonal contraception (EHC) contains progestogen only.
- It is more effective at preventing pregnancy the earlier it is taken.
- It is licensed to be taken up to 72 hours after a single episode of unprotected sex but may given up to 120 hours.
- It is available from pharmacies and contraceptive providers.
- Consider a copper IUD if maximum effectiveness is a priority.

Available from nurses, doctors, and over-the-counter from pharmacists, the emergency pill—known as 'Levonelle®', containing LNG 1500 mcg—is often called the 'morning-after pill'. This name is unhelpful because, although it works better the earlier it is taken, it can also be started *much later* than the next morning after unprotected sex—up to 72 hours (sometimes even 120 hours) later.

The other method, which is to have a copper IUD fitted, works up to 5 days after unprotected sex or 5 days after the earliest time you could have released an egg. Having that is obviously more uncomfortable and a bit of a hassle, but the IUD method is definitely the more effective of the two and there can be other reasons to choose it (see below).

Either treatment could be necessary because of a contraceptive 'accident'—a condom rupturing or slipping off, for instance; or of course by being a 'late restarter' of the pill on top of the usual 7-day break; or because no method of contraception has been used, perhaps because of alcohol, drugs, or in some cases rape. It acts mainly by stopping egg release, but sometimes by preventing implantation (see Chapter 2). Most experts consider that it is not causing an abortion, though others may disagree (see Appendix 3 for discussion of some ethical aspects).

How effective is EHC?

In any group of women requesting emergency contraception(EC), many would not conceive anyway. If taken within 24 hours of the (earliest) unprotected sex it will prevent more than nine out of 10 (95 per cent) of the pregnancies that would have been conceived without EC. If taken later, between 48 and 72 hours, EC should prevent more than half (58 per cent) of the conceptions.

As the hormone method can sometimes work by just *delaying* egg release, not stopping it altogether, it is vital to use a method such as the condom right through until the next period starts, sometimes longer when a new method takes some days to become effective.

Tell the nurse or doctor if you are taking an enzyme-inducing drug (see Chapter 14), including St John's Wort. You should either take *two* tablets to compensate for the EHC being weakened, or to be extra safe you might choose to have a copper IUD fitted (see below)—even if it is not going to be your long-term method.

Who can't take EHC?

There are very few women who cannot take EHC. Exclusion includes women who:

- Are already pregnant.
- Have past history of serious allergy to any ingredients of the tablets (incredibly rare).
- Have a particular rare illness called acute porphyria.

What are the side-effects?

Mainly nausea (15 per cent), with vomiting in about 1–2 per cent of women. If a dose is vomited back within 2 hours it should be replaced. Continued vomiting may be a reason to use the IUD method instead.

What if EHC fails?

If your next period seems normal in length and heaviness, it is unlikely that you will be pregnant. But EHC can certainly fail, in about 1–3 per cent of cases treated overall, more if the risk was taken around ovulation and the treatment is started only after fertilization, or if other risks were taken earlier in the cycle. If the method fails the EC pills have not been shown to harm a developing baby. Additionally, if there is already a pregnancy, the hormone treatment has not been shown to cause an abortion.

What follow-up is needed?

If you are worried, seek advice, but follow-up is usually only if you need it for your ongoing contraception (to see how the pill is suiting, and sometimes to remove a copper IUD if that was put in only to deal with the emergency situation). But you should always return 3–4 weeks later:

- If this is recommended in your case.
- If your next period is more than 7 days overdue or is exceptionally light.

◆ After 'quick starts' (see Chapter 11).

◆ If you get any abdominal pain. Always report this straight away: the method cannot cause an ectopic pregnancy, but it will not always prevent one in women who have got damaged tubes, something they can have without being aware of it.

Do I need to take the emergency pill if I've missed some COC or POP pills?

With the ordinary combined pill, many people think the most risky time is mid-packet, when actually that is the best time to miss pills if you must do so! Almost the only time you need to get this emergency after-sex treatment is if you have been more than 48 hours *late restarting a packet after your pill-free week, or have missed two or more pills in the first week of a pack*. See Chapter 13 for more details; also Chapter 17 for the advice which applies if you miss POP tablets.

You should take your next regular pill when it is due, and will also need to use an extra method such as condoms or avoid sex until your combined pill or POP is effective again (7 or 2 days, respectively).

When might inserting a copper IUD be recommended instead?

The main reasons are:

1. When you want the most effective method there is—and are prepared to handle the discomfort and potential problems of IUD insertion.

2. When it is:

   ◆ More than 72 hours but not yet 5 days after any unprotected sex **or**

   ◆ Five days after the earliest time you could have released an egg, when this has been carefully and in good faith calculated by the doctor, working from information from you about your usual cycle lengths. This can make it possible to do something when other risks were also taken earlier in the cycle.

3. When you are vomiting so much you wouldn't be able to keep down the tablets.

4 Because you actually want a copper IUD anyway as your long-term method. Putting one in will then solve both your immediate and your longer-term family-planning problem.

If the IUD is not your choice for the long term, it can also be removed after the next period, having dealt with the immediate crisis. You could wait until a new method, such as an injection, implant, or pill is fully effective first. Alternatively, if you have very heavy or painful periods your IUD could be exchanged for an IUS—but, unfortunately, the IUS should not itself be used directly in this emergency way.

19

The male pill

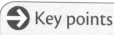 **Key points**

♦ Male contraception is biologically more difficult than female contraception.

♦ Vasectomy is the only male method currently available that doesn't require something to be done at the time of sex.

♦ Research is focusing on future methods that act to either stop sperm production, inactivate sperm, or block sperm release.

Women, would you ever trust a man who said he was on the male pill?

Despite that fact that the only contraceptive choices for men are withdrawal, condoms, or vasectomy, male contraception actually accounts for almost one-third of contraceptive use in many countries. The male pill has long been in development and continues to be queried because of its scientific complexity and questions about its cultural acceptance. The latter focuses on the debate of whether or not men can be trusted to take a contraceptive pill—after all, it's not them who have to carry the baby!

Yet surveys repeatedly indicate that men are willing to use a male contraceptive if it were available. Perhaps more importantly, 98 per cent of women in stable relationships would be willing to rely on their male partner to use contraception.

Research into male methods

Male contraception is biologically more difficult to achieve than female contraception. The main reason is that there is no single regular event like egg release which can be stopped. The manufacture of sperm is a continuous process throughout a man's life, from puberty to death. So instead of just stopping one egg being released about 13 times a year, we have to interfere with a process producing 1000–2000 sperm a second—hundreds of millions of them every time a man ejaculates.

Secondly, just as in the woman, any pill must not affect libido, must give extremely good protection against pregnancy, and be as free as possible from side-effects. There is a special risk here too that interference with the production of the sperm might be incomplete. So if one sperm were to be *damaged* by whatever the treatment might be, yet managed to fertilize an egg, this might result in the birth of an abnormal baby.

Another problem is that the manufacturing process takes a long time, about 70 days in the human male. Thus any male pill working on the manufacturing process will take at least 2 months to become effective. It also means that there must be a long recovery period after stopping the method. After some of the experimental methods have been stopped, more than the usual number of abnormal sperm has been seen. So if in the recovery period another method of family planning were inadequately used, again there is the fear of an increased risk of adverse effects on the baby.

Stopping sperm production

The pituitary gland of a man produces the same two hormones that are important in the menstrual cycle, namely FSH and LH. In a man, FSH is directly involved to promote sperm manufacture. LH, on the other hand, stimulates special cells, also in the testicle, which produce the male hormone, testosterone. This hormone, as well as producing the special sexual characteristics of a man such as the deepening of his voice, the hairiness of his chin, and his sex drive, joins with FSH in the business of manufacturing normal fertile sperm. So, if the levels of FSH and LH reaching the testicles can be made to drop, the process of sperm manufacture will cease. Clinical trials have used an injection plus implant to deliver a combination of a *progestogen with an androgen*, an artificial equivalent of testosterone. This blocks both pituitary hormones, and so switches off the man's own testosterone, while the androgen from the contraceptive maintains his libido. Although initially promising, the results so far are variable: it does not stop sperm production completely in every man, and there are side-effects (e.g. increased acne spots).

Other methods being researched include using a synthetic blocking drug to stop the man's GnRH, which is pulsed from the hypothalamus to the pituitary gland to release both FSH and LH. Another molecule of interest is *inhibin* (Fig. 19.1). This only suppresses FSH and should not affect the LH which controls a man's own testosterone production.

Drugs can also disrupt sperm production. One of these, *gossypol*, first discovered in cottonseed oil in China, has undergone extensive research: but there continue to be concerns about unwanted side-effects and also lack of reversibility.

Inactivating or blocking sperm

One idea has been to inactivate the mature sperm, which would enable more rapid loss and return of fertility than by any of the methods above, which interfere with sperm manufacture. Vaccination against GnRH and FSH has been suggested, causing men to develop immunity against their own sperm. Alternatively, sperm

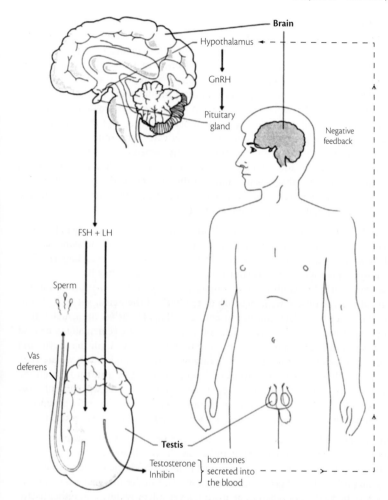

Figure 19.1 How reproductive hormones work in men.
Note: testosterone, as well as having well-known effects as an androgen, can suppress FSH and LH. Inhibin feeds back to suppress FSH alone.

could be blocked from reaching the fluid that a man ejaculates. He would still ejaculate about the same amount of sperm-supporting fluid, so this would be like reversible vasectomy—indeed various kinds of taps and removable blocks in the vas have also been tried, so far without a practical outcome.

But currently the most promising method of this type is the *'dry orgasm male pill'* . . .. It is based on a highly unusual side-effect happening in users of two drugs that have been around a long time: thioridazine is a sedative and phenoxybenzamine is used to treat a rare form of raised blood pressure. Back in 1961, a medical research paper was published in the USA with a most unusual title: 'Thioridazine-induced inhibition of masturbatory ejaculation in an adolescent'. This means that a young man had reported to his psychiatrist that when he masturbated he was dry, didn't produce any fluid at all . . . yet importantly he still liked to do it, having the same sensations as he used to have before starting that treatment. The other drug (phenyoxybenzamine) was later tried out in Israel for its contraceptive effect. At no time while on treatment did any of the 13 volunteers produce any semen at all at ejaculation, yet their semen volume and quality became normal again within a day or two of stopping. Just as for thioridazine, none of the men noticed any bad effects on their libido, erection, sexual performance, or on their sensations of orgasm and ejaculation—despite no fluid being emitted.

Since then two pharmacologists, Amobi and Smith at King's College in London, have systematically tested both these drugs and others with the same 'chemical signature'—using bits of vas excised from volunteers at the Margaret Pyke (London) and Elliot-Smith (Oxford) vasectomy clinics. They have discovered how they work: by paralysing the longitudinal (up and down) muscles in the walls of the vas tube system right up to the back of the penis, yet still permitting the other (circular) muscles to contract. This abolishes the usual sort of 'Mexican wave' down the vas, which normally propels the semen along: instead there is a sphincter action, reversibly stopping the flow of both the sperm and all the supporting seminal fluid. Working with Amobi and Smith we are now seeking funding to take this promising contraceptive forward, through all the required phases of clinical testing for efficacy and safety. This will certainly cost millions of dollars and take at least 10 more years, meaning sadly around 60 years since those first reports before a practical male pill can be marketed . . ..

This kind of pill has great potential to be taken pre-coitally, so a woman might supervise her partner swallowing it and know she would be safe when they later had sex . . .. Or instead (like the hormonal male methods mentioned earlier) the drug might be released gradually from an implant under the man's skin, allowing sex to be more spontaneous, at any time, yet still providing that rather useful visual confirmation of his claim to be protected!

Conclusion

Apart from withdrawal, the condom and vasectomy remain the only practical male methods available now, and for the near future. Whether or not the pharmaceutical industry will consider male contraception to be a worthwhile investment carries a major question mark in the present economic climate. And we guess that the whole subject of acceptability by the male consumers and especially by their female partners will continue to be debated, for many years to come!

20

Postscript

Young people, sex and the pill

Young people coming to a GP, family-planning doctor or nurse for advice should be met where they are at, no pressure. Most are already having sex, they want and they should definitely get contraceptive advice and supplies (see below), in confidence and completely non-judgmentally.

That said, it is just a factual statement, telling it how it is, that *one* of the *options* for a teenager – along with the various contraceptive options which include the pill - is "saving sex" i.e. not having it yet! (with this person or at all maybe, until they are sure they have met 'Mr or Miss Right'). Who can doubt that, medically, this is a very safe path to tread? In fact, it is the only one with a zero risk of STIs and since method-failures can't happen, no unwanted conceptions - plus very probably less psychological trauma during subsequent teenage years through likely multiple "bust-ups". Yet it is not an option to mention unless the person advising is sure it is appropriate to do so. Reminding her at an opportune moment of her right to choose this path might, for example, be really helpful for a teenager who feels pressurized by her boyfriend, or by peer pressure from girlfriends. But this is a choice for her (or it could be him) to make, not one to be pushed - whether by parents or anyone else.

Let's face it, ours is a society where most young people receive little guidance, and plenty of bad examples from unhelpful role models, like some 'Celebs'. Society has largely thrown out old values and in the words of Gladys Mwiti, a Tear Fund worker in Nairobi, *'You cannot fill a values vacuum with condoms.'* Furthermore, concerned as they rightly are with harm reduction, to prevent unplanned pregnancies and abortions and the spread of STIs, school-teachers, doctors and nurses can sometimes - without meaning to - come over as giving an official seal of approval for ever younger teenage sex.

As the sexologist Dr Esther Sapire wrote in her book *Contraception and Sexuality in Health and Disease* (McGraw-Hill):

> *Sex is part of oneself to accept and live with comfortably and enjoy.*
> *It is not something that comes in from outside and takes over the body*
> *and flies off. It is something we* **are** *not [just] something we* **do** *as a*
> *physical act, and it cannot be isolated from the total relationship. Sex*
> *is an expression of love, and is only one aspect of it which enhances the*

> *relationship.... There is a time when one is ready for sexual experiences, but if the process is hastened unduly without allowing the natural process to 'unfold' at its own pace, it may never function well .... like a closed, exquisite rosebud being pulled open by someone impatient to see it in its fully glory—only to find the petals bruised and torn in the process....*

Many people have discovered that for themselves, and also that making love is usually best when it's with a person who has become your "best mate" of the opposite sex - and on the first date how likely is it you can know that? Responsible sex means positive answers to three questions before making love: 'Do we want, and can we care for, a baby?'; 'if not, are we using a reliable method of family planning, such as the Pill, with a condom also as needed for safer sex?'; and, often forgotten, 'Will making love with this person lead to anyone, my partner, myself, or any third party, being hurt?

Yet, we agree completely that those who say (particularly in America) that "abstinence education" is all that young people should get must be living on another planet! However much it (abstinence) might be "best" – meaning medically safest - it's unrealistic for many people, given the power of our sex hormones ... not to mention alcohol.... And it's been shown not to work, even in America. So let's not let the 'best' become the enemy of the "good". What's that? Well in my opinion it's not "sex education"! Words matter: saying "sex education" can be unhelpful, you often get the response from journalists and others that this is "educating them to do sex". Some even seem to believe against all the evidence that "if only you didn't tell them they wouldn't do it". So we prefer people to call it "sex and relationships education" (SRE for short), not only to minimise those silly responses but also because that's what it should always be, anyway: top quality SRE for boys as well as girls.

This should start (ideally) from as young as about age three onwards by good parenting, basically just answering a child's questions in an unembarrassed and age-appropriate way. *Then they become teenagers!...* No debate, it is always mighty difficult to be a good parent with respect to issues of sex and drugs – but both teens and their parents can get a lot of help through the excellent website www.parentlineplus.org.uk Good SRE should continue at school and contraceptives supplied as and when needed, (whether at a dedicated young persons' clinic, GP surgery or pharmacy), including emergency contraception (the morning-after pill) and condoms for STI prevention. Confidentiality is crucial: it must be real but it must also have the "feel" of being real to the young person, whoever they speak with - from Reception staff onwards. Very importantly, as one group of youngsters said in a Focus group, when asked who would be the best provider of their own contraception: "someone with a smile would be your best bet!" (Meaning, regrettably, that they had met with providers who were unsmiling and probably not very sympathetic either).

Other excellent websites are:

> www.ruthinking.co.uk [User-friendly, packed with information
> and makes it really easy for young people to access services].

> www.likeitis.org.uk [Gives young people "a chance to get sexual
> health information exactly like it is - no frills & no judgments..."]

What about the Pill (or other chosen contraception, since actually the more "forgettable" methods like the injection or an implant are often better choices for teens), in all this? It cannot be expected to be a cure-all of society's ills. Neither should it be blamed for too many of them—they are caused by people, not by the Pill. Certainly it can enable some people to behave irresponsibly, people who forget that bodies also have feelings and emotions attached. Even then, at least a disastrous pregnancy will be avoided. A child has the best chance in life if born to parents who trust each other and because of their commitment are prepared to keep *working* on their relationship, so as to ensure an emotionally secure and happy home for all the years he or she needs to reach maturity. *And then* the Pill and other methods can help that home not to be overwhelmed by more new arrivals than the family, or the family's country and indeed as we now appreciate, their world, can properly care for!

John Guillebaud & Anne MacGregor

May 2009

Glossary

abortion the end of a pregnancy at any time before independent life is possible. Abortion may be spontaneous (a miscarriage) or induced by an operation or prescribed medication. Doctors often use the term 'termination of pregnancy' (TOP) instead

androgenic masculinizing, the effect of an androgen such as testosterone

BMI (body mass index) this is the *weight* of a person in kilograms divided by *height* in metres squared. It gives the best measure of being overweight (or underweight) as related to one's height. The normal range of BMI is 19–25

BTB (breakthrough bleeding) any unexpected bleeding on the combined pill happening on tablet-taking days, between the hormone-withdrawal bleeds ('periods')

cervix the narrow lower end of the *uterus*, containing the entrance to it. Sometimes called 'the neck of the womb'

chlamydia the most common cause of STI of the fallopian tubes, also known as salpingitis or pelvic infection, with pelvic pain as a possible symptom. Sometimes it causes 'BTB' in pill takers. It can lead to ectopic pregnancies or sterility, through damaged or blocked fallopian tubes. Importantly, it can be 'silent', without symptoms

chloasma (also known as **melasma**) abnormal facial skin pigmentation occurring in some women during pregnancy or when taking the combined pill

COC (combined oral contraceptive) taken by mouth and which contains two hormones: one a *progestogen* and the other an *oestrogen*. Usually called the pill

cone biopsy a minor operation under general anaesthesia to remove some skin at the entrance to the uterus in order to treat some abnormal cells found by cervical smear. Abnormal cells are now more often removed with a so-called 'large loop', as an out-patient under local anaesthetic

contraception prevention of pregnancy by a reversible method. This definition excludes the other two types of birth control, which are sterilization and abortion

contraceptive any substance or device which reversibly prevents conception (while allowing intercourse)

contraindications medical reasons to avoid a contraceptive

corpus luteum the yellow body formed in the ovary during the menstrual cycle from the largest follicle, after it has released its egg

cystitis inflammation of the urinary bladder, usually caused by infection, provoking a desire to pass urine more frequently and often a burning sensation on doing so

D&C (dilatation and curettage) with hysteroscopy a common minor operation when a narrow scope and/or a curette is passed into the uterus through the *cervix*. The inside of the uterus is looked at, tissue can be taken for laboratory examination (see also *endometrial biopsy*), or it can be completely emptied, e.g. after a miscarriage or induced abortion which has been incomplete

EE (ethinylestradiol) the main artificial oestrogen used in the pill, not to be confused with the natural oestrogen used in HRT

ectopic pregnancy a pregnancy in the wrong place, i.e. anywhere other than in the uterus. The most common site is in the uterine (fallopian) tube. An urgent operation is necessary, because the growing pregnancy can cause internal bleeding. The tubes have often been damaged by a previous pelvic infection, usually from chlamydia

ejaculation the spurting-out of semen (ejaculate) from the penis when a man has a climax

embolism transfer in the bloodstream of a mass, such as a blood clot from a vein, to lodge elsewhere, generally in the lungs (pulmonary embolism)

embryo name given to the early pregnancy from fertilization for the first 8 weeks (then called the *fetus*)

endometrium the special lining of the uterus, which is prepared by the hormones of the menstrual cycle in readiness for implantation of an embryo— or otherwise shed at the menstrual period

fertilization the union of sperm and egg cell. The fertilized egg divides to produce an embryo

fetus name for any growing baby after 8 weeks of intrauterine life

fimbriae the fringe-like fronds which surround the outer end of each uterine tube

follicle a small fluid-filled balloon-like structure in the ovary, containing an egg cell

FSH (follicle-stimulating hormone) the hormone produced by the pituitary gland, which stimulates the growth of follicles in the ovary and which in turn produce oestrogen and the maturing of an egg cell in the largest follicle

GnRH (gonadotrophin-releasing hormone) the hormone produced by the *hypothalamus*, which travels to the pituitary gland causing the release of *FSH* and *LH* into the bloodstream

GUM (genitourinary medicine) the branch of medicine specializing in treating *STIs*

hCG (human chorionic gonadotrophin) the hormone produced by an early pregnancy, which travels to the ovary in the bloodstream and causes its corpus luteum to continue producing oestrogen and progesterone beyond the usual 14 days

HIV/AIDS human immunodeficiency virus/the sexually transmissible cause of acquired immune deficiency syndrome, which without treatment leads to lack of immune resistance to infections and death

hormone a chemical substance produced in one organ and carried in the bloodstream like a 'chemical messenger' to another organ or tissue, whose function it influences or alters

HRT (hormone replacement therapy) treatment with *natural* oestrogen, often along with a progestogen, given when women lack sufficient from their own ovaries, e.g. after the menopause

hypertension high blood pressure, above the accepted normal level

hysterectomy an operation to remove the uterus

hypothalamus the structure at the base of the brain which releases *GnRH*

implantation the process of the embedding of the developing embryo in the *endometrium*

IUD (intrauterine device) a small plastic device, which usually carries copper in the form of wire or bands and is inserted into the uterus to prevent pregnancy

IUS (intrauterine system) a small plastic device slowly releasing a *hormone*, currently always a *progestogen*, into the uterus to prevent pregnancy

LH (luteinizing hormone) the hormone produced by the pituitary gland that causes egg release, and the production and maintenance of the corpus luteum

libido the internal drive and urge of the sexual instinct

lipids fats and associated chemical substances, carried in the blood

menopause cessation of the menstrual periods due to failure of ovulation and hormone production by the ovaries. Often used inaccurately for the climacteric or the perimenopause time, which is several years before and after periods actually cease

menstrual cycle the cycle of hormone and other changes in a woman's body which leads to a regular discharge of blood from the non-pregnant uterus

mestranol an artificial oestrogen, now rarely used

monophasic combined pills containing a fixed dose of ethinylestradiol and progestogen

mucus such as cervical mucus, a slippery fluid produced by the glands of the cervix. Progestogens change it so that it impedes sperm when they try to enter the uterus

oestrogen the female sex hormone produced by the ovary throughout the menstrual cycle

oestrogen-dominant pill a combined pill whose biological effects on the body are due to the relatively stronger effect of the oestrogen it contains than to the progestogen

ovary the female sex gland in which ova (egg cells) are developed and which is the main source of natural sex hormones

ovulation release of the ovum or ova from the ovary—more often called egg release in this book

PCOS (polycystic ovary syndrome) a condition in which multiple small cysts develop around the outside of the ovary and the woman has *androgenic* effects such as acne or unwanted hair growth

phasic combined pills containing two (biphasic) or three (triphasic) different doses of ethinylestradiol and progestogen

phlebitis thrombosis and inflammation involving a vein—usually a superficial vein of the leg—which causes it to become hard and very tender

pituitary gland the gland, about the size of a pea, on a stalk at the base of the brain, which produces many important hormones including *FSH* and *LH*

POP (progestogen-only pill) as the name suggests, a pill with only the one hormone present, an artificial progestogen. Is even safer than the COC, since it is EE-free

progesterone the other main sex hormone produced by the ovaries (see *oestrogen*). This hormone is produced only in the second half of the menstrual cycle, by the corpus luteum. It prepares the body, especially the uterus, for pregnancy. It is one of the general class of progestogens

progestogen a number of artificial progestogens that are chemically related to natural *progesterone*

progestogen-dominant pill a combined pill whose biological effects on the body are due more to the relatively higher dose of progestogen it contains than to the oestrogen

prolactin a hormone produced by the pituitary gland which stimulates the breasts to produce milk and is also involved in the menstrual cycle

prostaglandins natural substances manufactured and released within many tissues of the body. Some natural prostaglandins cause the uterus to contract, and these and other artificial variants can therefore be used to cause an induced abortion

puberty the time when a boy or girl begins to develop secondary sex characteristics and then becomes fertile. In a girl, the most significant event is the onset of periods, correctly called the menarche

pyridoxine vitamin B_6

spermicide a substance which is capable of killing sperm

sterilization an operation in a person of either sex which permanently prevents pregnancy, and which is either impossible or difficult to reverse

STIs (sexually transmitted infections) there are many of these, including *chlamydia*—usually best treated at a GUM clinic

thrombosis the formation of a blood clot within a blood vessel (artery or vein). Arterial thrombosis can produce *heart attacks* or *strokes*; venous thrombosis in the legs can spread to the lungs to cause *pulmonary embolism*

uterine (fallopian) tubes the tubes which in the female convey the egg to the uterus, and within which fertilization by a sperm usually occurs

uterus (womb) the hollow organ in which a pregnancy develops

vagina the distensible passageway which extends from the cervix to the vulva, into which the penis is inserted during intercourse

vas deferens the tube in the male which conveys the sperm from the epididymis to the base of the penis. It is the tube that is divided at *vasectomy*

vasectomy male sterilization

vulva the name given to the female external genital structures

WTB (withdrawal bleeding) bleeding from the uterus caused by the woman herself when she stops the supply of hormones to it, by taking a break at the end of each packet as (usually) instructed. It occurs during the *pill-free interval*.

Appendix 1

Top tips for pill takers

1. Read your FPA information leaflet and keep it safe, for ongoing reference. If you do lose it, you can read the information on line at http://www.fpa.org.uk.

2. Say to yourself over and over: 'I must never be a late restarter'... (Chapter 13). This is because the pill-free interval (PFI) is a time when your ovaries are not getting any effect from the pill hormones and might be beginning to 'wake up'—extending this time risks pregnancy.

3. Sex during the 7 days after any packet is only safe if you do go on to the next one: otherwise (if you are stopping the method for any reason), start using a method such as condoms after the last pill in the pack.

4. Even if your 'period' (WTB) has not stopped yet, never start your next packet late.

5. If you're afraid you might forget to start a new pack, ask for an ED pack, which has 'dummy' pills to take during the 'pill-free' week.

6. The pill only works if you take it correctly: with any type of packaging, each new pack will always start on the same day of the week.

7. Even if bleeding (BTB) during tablet taking is like a 'period', carry on pill taking.

8. Nausea is a common early symptom. Both BTB and nausea usually settle as your body gets used to the pill.

9. Know what to do if any pill(s) are more than 24 hours late (see Chapter 13).

10. Other things that may stop the pill from working include vomiting (within 2 hours) and some drugs (Chapter 14).

11. See a doctor at once if you have serious side-effects (Chapter 15).

12. To avoid 'periods' (withdrawal bleeds) at weekends: as a one-off, you only need to shorten one PFI (Chapter 12).

13. You can usually avoid all bleeding on holidays, etc., by running packs together. Discuss this with whoever provides your pills if you want to continue missing out 'periods' long term, e.g. tricycling or taking the pill continuously 365/365 (Chapter 12).

14. Good though it is as a contraceptive, the pill does not give adequate protection against chlamydia and the other STIs. Whenever in doubt, especially with a new partner, use a condom as well.

15. Finally, always feel free to telephone or contact your pill-provider or the FPA helpline (0845 122 8690) for any reasons of your own, including any symptoms you would like dealt with. Thereafter there are really only three key things to be checked on at follow-ups visits for the pill:

   ◆ Blood pressure.
   ◆ Headaches and migraine.
   ◆ Troublesome side-effects, new diseases, or risk factors that affect you taking the pill.

Appendix 2

What is the ideal contraceptive?

What should we look for, anyway, in a method of birth control, present or future? Box A2.1 provides a useful checklist of what would be ideal. Items 1–5 are all vitally important things to aim for.

Box A2.1 Features of the ideal contraceptive

1. 100 per cent effective.
2. 100 per cent safe, with no unwanted effects—both risky and nuisance-type.
3. 100 per cent reversible.
4. Convenient, independent of intercourse.
5. Effective after acceptable, simple, painless procedures(s), not relying on the user's memory, i.e. fully 'forgettable'.
6. Reversed by a simple, painless process under the user's control.
7. Cheap, based on simple technology, easy to distribute.
8. Independent of the medical profession.
9. Acceptable to every culture, religion, and political view.
10. Used by, or obviously visible to, the woman.
11. Giving one or more non-contraceptive beneficial side-effects, such as reduced menstrual problems and protection against STIs, particularly HIV/AIDS.

It would be great if we didn't have to add number 10 to the list. It is a sad comment on the relationship of many couples that they can sleep together yet be unable to trust each other. More specifically, a lot of *men* are not trustworthy about contraception, or are just forgetful or careless. Either partner can be unreliable, of course, but only the woman ends up pregnant. An advantage of the condom is that it gives visual proof that it has in fact been effectively used.

Perhaps the last item is asking for too much, but we *are* talking about the ideal. For all its faults, the pill does help women who suffer discomfort or misery from their so-called 'normal' menstrual cycles. A method which was ideal in all the other ways listed in Box A2.1, such as a simple, painless, totally reversible method of female sterilization, might still leave some women less well off than on the pill, if they continued to have heavy, painful periods, premenstrual tension, and the like.

Figure A2.1 illustrates the various stages or events in reproduction at which birth control methods either do now, or could one day, operate. The main points were described in Chapter 2.

Any method developed has to be based on detecting or interfering with one of these stages. It is a complex system, so it is never going to be easy to alter it without the possibility of unwanted spin-offs and side-effects. This means expensive testing. Understandable caution plus fears about litigation have made development of new methods so expensive and prolonged (15 years is the minimum) as to tend to stop it altogether.

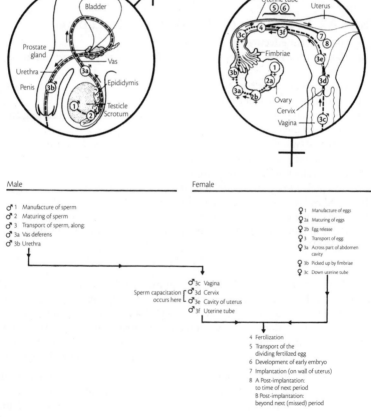

Figure A2.1 The stages of reproduction.

Appendix 3

Some ethical aspects of contraception

A question which concerns some people is whether methods which are able to act after fertilization are in reality abortifacients (causing an abortion) and hence ethically unacceptable. We take the view that methods that sometimes work after fertilization (see Chapter 2) but before the completion of implantation are not causing abortions. Why do we see these as correctly in the category of contraceptive methods?

A complication for the debate is that when a woman uses a method that can prevent pregnancy in more than one way, such as the POP: did it prevent a possible pregnancy by stopping ovulation or by preventing the sperm from getting through to the egg, or was it by interfering later with the fertilized egg or embryo (which is believed to be a much weaker action with the POP, but still might be how it worked when the others failed)?

A most important point is that the fact that a method is *capable* of working in a post-fertilization way does not mean it necessarily ever needs to do so. Thus women who are conscientious COC pill takers, never once lengthening their pill-free week even by an hour, or users of Depo-Provera®, never being late with their next 12-weekly dose, can be confident that their avoidance of pregnancy is entirely due to the block to ovulation (egg release) and also to the mucus block to sperm. Those mechanisms are so strong that the back-up by blocking implantation will never be needed, even during years of use.

The question 'could my method be causing an induced miscarriage/abortion?' therefore only arises with methods that do not, or do not always, prevent egg release, i.e. only the intrauterine methods, all the POPs, and of course with EC. Like most healthcare professionals, we consider that the answer is still 'no' in all these cases even if they might, rarely or sometimes, operate by a pre-implantation but post-fertilization mechanism. But that depends on definitions, and specifically on accepting the definition of 'conception' as only being complete after implantation.

Let's go back to basics. See Chapter 2. After any fertilization there is cell division to produce the earliest embryo, a fluid-filled sac known as the blastocyst. This reaches the uterus and begins to stick to its wall (implant) about 5 days after fertilization. It makes hCG and only if it implants successfully can this enter the mother's bloodstream and prevent the regular failure of the corpus luteum, and the resultant inevitable loss of the blastocyst in the next menstrual flow.

So what is the status of this unimplanted blastocyst? Clearly while it is free in the uterine cavity it still has 100 per cent '*no go*' status. It is a certainty, that in a few days it is going to be flushed through the cervix and vagina in a gush of debris and blood (the menses).

This 'no go' status can only change to 'go' after implantation allows the crucial hCG signal to get back via the bloodstream to the mother's active ovary. This tells its corpus luteum to continue to produce essential oestrogen and progesterone, to maintain the uterine lining and so prevent the next period. Three things follow from this:

- First, until then it has no more chance of life than the particular sperm and egg that made it, about 5 days earlier, in the tube. Thereafter, it has about an 80 per cent chance of making it to term.
- Secondly, until implantation there is no proper two-way **relationship** with the mother.
- Thirdly, best estimates suggest that up to 50 per cent of blastocysts fail to implant. Isn't it common sense not to assign the importance, respect, and care to this entity, with which nature is so prodigal, as most of us rightly give to the fetus later, after implantation?

If these three points are accepted, abortion would only be when the pregnancy is stopped after that implantation time, when there is both a relationship with the mother and for the first time there are above-zero prospects of going on to term.

From these considerations one can write an equation for the definition of conception as follows:

CONCEPTION = FERTILIZATION + IMPLANTATION

(being with child)   (crucial)   (also crucial)

To summarize, if you accept the equation above that is based on the science of Chapter 2, you can agree wholeheartedly with those who say that '*life begins at conception*'—you just don't see that as being simultaneous with fertilization. The equation makes it justifiable to use methods of contraception that might sometimes block implantation. This is also the UK legal position, established finally in 2002 by the Judicial Review on EC.

Appendix 4

Useful contacts

http://www.fpa.org.uk: comes first, because so often all you need can be accessed here, or you can find out by phoning their superb Helpline—0845 122 8690. The FPA specializes in client/user information generally, including essential leaflets on all the methods—and on many related subjects such as STIs and abortion. Can also tell you how to access locally, near where you live, appropriate (for your problem) sexual and reproductive health.

http://www.brook.org.uk: similar to the FPA in some ways, but mainly for the under-25s. Has a secure on-line enquiry service and a free Helpline: 0800 0185023.

http://www.margaretpyke.org: the Margaret Pyke Centre is the hub of a network of busy open-access clinics in central London (appointments line: 020 7530 3650) and its charitable Trust supports contraceptive training and research (volunteers welcome!).

http://www.ippf.org.uk: online version of the Directory of Hormonal Contraception, with names of equivalent pill brands and other hormonal contraceptives as used throughout the world.

http://www.fertilityuk.org: the fertility awareness and NFP service, including teachers available locally.

http://www.ruthinking.co.uk: a highly user-friendly website that fully informs, plus makes it really easy for young people to access services: with a good search engine giving details of their local clinics, for both contraception and sexual health with testing and treatment for STIs. Supported by the Teenage Pregnancy Unit.

http://www.likeitis.org: 'What likeitis does is give young people a chance to get sexual health information exactly like it is: with no frills, no judgements and definitely no holds barred' (Marie Stopes International).

http://www.sexplained.com: slogan is 'From the clinic to the street'. Very frank and accessible website for young people.

http://www.teenagehealthfreak.com: brilliant comprehensive health website. FAQs as asked by teenagers, on all health subjects, not just reproductive health—from anorexia to zits!

http://www.fsrh.org: primarily for healthcare professionals, this includes Faculty of Sexual and Reproductive Healthcare's Guidance PDFs about each method of contraception and other authoritative reports.

http://www.who.int/reproductive-health: WHO's Eligibility Criteria and new Practice Recommendations for healthcare professionals, and informed lay persons, worldwide.

Appendix 5

Further reading

For more information about *all* methods of contraception:

Szarewski A and Guillebaud J (2000). *Contraception: A User's Guide*. Oxford: Oxford University Press. Although some information is now out-dated, this book still provides useful guidance.

Other books which, although written primarily for healthcare professionals, are readily understandable and often used by general readers:

Glasier A and Gebbie A (2008). *Handbook of Family Planning and Reproductive Healthcare*, 5th edition. Edinburgh: Churchill Livingstone (Elsevier).

Guillebaud J (2007). *Contraception Today—A Pocketbook for Primary Care Practitioners*, 6th edition. London: Informa Healthcare.

Guillebaud J (2009). *Contraception—Your Questions Answered*, 5th edition. Edinburgh: Churchill Livingstone (Elsevier).

Miscellaneous, also relevant:

Cooper E and Guillebaud J (1999). *Sexuality and Disability*. Oxford: Radcliffe Medical Press.

Djerassi, C. (1981). *The Politics of Contraception: Birth Control in the Year 2001*. San Francisco: WH Freeman & Co.

Ehrlich P and Ehrlich A (1991). *The Population Explosion*. London: Arrow Books.

Skrine R and Montford H (2001). *Psychosexual Medicine—An Introduction*. London: Arnold Publishing.

Family Planning Association's (http://www.fpa.org.uk) own publications and excellent leaflets can be ordered through 0845 122 8600 or fpadirect@fpa.org.uk.

Appendix 5

Further reading

Index

Where headings and sub-headings are followed by several page references, those numbers in **bold italic** indicate a more extensive treatment of the topic.